Teaching Evidence-Based Medicine

Daniella A. Zipkin
Editor

Teaching Evidence-Based Medicine

A Toolkit for Educators

Springer

Editor
Daniella A. Zipkin
Department of Medicine
Duke University School of Medicine
Durham, NC, USA

ISBN 978-3-031-11173-0 ISBN 978-3-031-11174-7 (eBook)
https://doi.org/10.1007/978-3-031-11174-7

This Springer imprint is published by the registered company Springer Nature Switzerland AG
The registered company address is: Gewerbestrasse 11, 6330 Cham, Switzerland

Acknowledgments

The author team would like to thank Dr. Sheri Keitz for her indefatigable championing of evidence-based practice and for creating and nurturing the EBP teaching space where many of us met and continue to teach annually.

Contents

Contributors

Kathleen W. Bartlett Department of Pediatrics, Duke Children's Hospital, Duke University, Durham, NC, USA

Zackary D. Berger Division of General Internal Medicine, Department of Medicine, John Hopkins School of Medicine, Baltimore, MD, USA

Jeffrey Kushinka Department of Internal Medicine, Virginia Commonwealth University School of Medicine, Richmond, VA, USA

Deepa Rani Nandiwada Division of General Internal Medicine, Department of Medicine, Penn Center for Primary Care Penn Presbyterian Hospital, University of Pennsylvania Perelman School of Medicine, Philadelphia, PA, USA

Matthew Tuck Department of Medicine, Veterans Affairs Medical Center, Medical Service, George Washington University, Washington, DC, USA

Megan von Isenburg Medical Center Library, School of Medicine, Duke University, Durham, NC, USA

Daniella A. Zipkin Department of Medicine, Duke University Health System, Duke University School of Medicine, Durham, NC, USA

1 How To Use This Book

Matthew Tuck and Daniella A. Zipkin

Introduction

This book is designed as a resource to help health professions educators teach evidence-based medicine (EBM) principles and practice. Our aim is to provide material which is adaptable to learners of various backgrounds. Each chapter offers core EBM content along with tips for teaching that content with extensive examples, sample materials, and sample video tutorials. We share examples in different clinical domains throughout this book and all of our examples can be applied to diverse clinical scenarios with either undergraduate or graduate medical education audiences in various fields.

Before jumping into the content, it is critical to frame the learning experience intended for your learners. This chapter focuses on planning your own curriculum for your own environment, and we highly recommend using this chapter before the content chapters.

M. Tuck
Department of Medicine, Veterans Affairs Medical Center, Medical Service, George Washington University, Washington, DC, USA
e-mail: Matthew.Tuck@va.gov

D. A. Zipkin (✉)
Department of Medicine, Duke University Health System, Duke University School of Medicine, Durham, NC, USA
e-mail: daniella.zipkin@duke.edu

D. A. Zipkin (ed.), *Teaching Evidence-Based Medicine*,
https://doi.org/10.1007/978-3-031-11174-7_1

Background and Rationale for Evidence-Based Medicine Teaching

"Evidence based medicine is the conscientious, explicit and judicious use of current best evidence in making decisions about the care of individual patients. The practice of evidence-based medicine means integrating individual clinical expertise with the best available external clinical evidence from systematic research." [1] David Sackett introduced the term "critical appraisal" in 1981 in a series of articles designed to assist clinicians in interpreting research. He, along with others, published the foundational text "Clinical Epidemiology" in 1985, now in its third revision [2]. Sackett's colleague, Gordon Guyatt, first used the term "evidence based medicine" in an article in the ACP Journal Club in 1991 [3]. He first edited the core text "User's Guides to the Medical Literature" in 2002, which is now in its third edition [4].

EBM has become a frequently used phrase among physicians and medical institutions over the years. While the use of the phrase can be subject to interpretation and is sometimes controversial, as many things can be described as evidence, most clinicians are in agreement about the importance of reviewing and appraising the literature and applying it to the care of our patients. Skill in EBM is a part of the Practice-Based Learning and Improvement competency outlined by the Accreditation Council for Graduate Medical Education (ACGME), and is an expected component of graduate medical training [5]. The Liaison Committee on Medical Education (LCME) has similar expectations for medical students [6].

Practicing EBM requires a good working knowledge of information sources, an understanding of the hierarchy in quality of evidence, and a facility with certain core EBM concepts. Patients trust us to have assimilated information correctly, and benefit when we communicate the evidence to them in a fashion that's tailored to their needs. Medical students, residents, and fellows expect that their training will prepare them for these tasks. The teaching of EBM in medical training is widely variable. Some programs address EBM topics in forums such as morning report and journal club. Others develop EBM curricula of varying lengths and depths. In this chapter, we aim to present resources to guide the formation or expansion of EBM curricula.

We invite readers to outline their own course goals and objectives, course content and methods, and evaluation tools, and consider common barriers in the creation of their own curricula.

Steps in Building your EBM Curriculum [7]

1. Define the learners within your teaching setting. What is their level of experience with the material? How much clinical exposure do they have currently?
2. Define the teaching time frame and available faculty. How long will teaching sessions last and how frequently will they occur? Who will teach the sessions?
3. Conduct a needs assessment of your learners through surveys, focus groups, or written testing. Often times, there are competing interests between the needs of the learners (e.g., what they need to do to be successful evidence-based

practitioners) and the educational administration (e.g., what they need to do to perform well on standardized examinations).

4. Argue for the necessity of implementing your curriculum. Present your proposal to the stakeholders at your institution. You will inevitably need support of these stakeholders to establish meaningful and sustainable curricula.
5. Once you have approval to create a curriculum, start at the end: where do you expect your learners to be by the end of the curriculum? What should they be able to do as a result of the curriculum?
6. Write goals of the overall curriculum. Examples might be, "by the end of this curriculum, learners should be able to critically appraise a study." Curricula can be very broad, or very focused.
7. List the EBM content areas and objectives for the individual learning session(s). We suggest using behaviorally-based measurable objectives, such as Bloom's Taxonomy [8], so that you are then able to measurably assess the impact of your curriculum.
8. Outline the teaching methods you will use. Discussion with collaborators can help to refine the best ways to incorporate adult-learning principles into the teaching methods. Examples for engaging strategies that are in keeping with adult learning theory include team-based learning, small group work, and experiential learning.
9. Draft a teaching session based on the content, learning objectives and teaching methods you have chosen. Use the resources outlined in this book as you create your teaching sessions.
10. Assess the learners and your curriculum and revise the curriculum accordingly. In undergraduate medical education, assessments of the learner often take the form of multiple-choice questions or may be more creative. For example, the learner may have to perform an objective structured clinical exercise (OSCE), wherein they must perform a search on PubMed and briefly appraise an article that informs the care and management of a standardized patient. In graduate medical education, assessing the learner often includes evaluation of their competency with evidence-based practice in relation to patient care. Assessments of the curriculum are based on how well your learners are doing on the learner assessments and whether the curriculum's goals were achieved. Peer educators can also be a helpful resource when assessing the curriculum.

Sample Curricular Goals and Objectives

It is helpful to begin by defining goals and contrasting them with objectives. Goals are broad plans for what you want to achieve, the general direction you're headed. Objectives are more specific actions you will take to reach the goals. Objectives should be written with a verb—ask yourself, "what will learners be able to DO when this teaching session is complete?"

Table 1.1 provides some sample goals and objectives for different course lengths and learner levels. They are intended as suggestions and guides to get you started, so that you can write your own!

Table 1.1 Sample goals and objectives by learner and course type

Course Length	Learner Level	Goals [This course will…]	Objectives [Learners will be able to…]
Short course	Novice (MS, PGY-1)	• Introduce the language of EBM • Illustrate question formation, study selection, and the hierarchy of evidence • Introduce core EBM definitions for different types of clinical questions • Highlight sources of bias in studies • Provide resources and references for critical appraisal and model several examples	• List the components of a well-structured question • Name the best study design for a clinical question • Identify sources of bias in studies on diagnostic testing and therapy • Calculate absolute risk reduction, relative risk reduction, number needed to treat • Interpret confidence intervals and describe their relationship to precision • List resources for evidence-based critical appraisal
	Inter-mediate (PGY-2)	• Enhance skills of question formation and study selection • Improve knowledge and skills involved in critical appraisal • Understand the process of diagnostic testing • Improve ability to detect and assess the impact of bias on study conclusions • Hone the selection of best published research evidence • Improve skills related to presentation of articles	• Articulate a focused clinical question • Identify high quality papers through electronic literature search • List and define critical appraisal criteria for major study types • Define pretest probability and describe how it is generated • Define likelihood ratio and state its utility in diagnostic testing • Explain how lead and length time bias can affect studies of screening • Define risk ratios, odds ratios, and hazard ratios, risk reductions, and number needed to treat • Succinctly present an article with assessment of its validity
	Advanced (PGY-3, fellow, faculty)	• Teach critical appraisal and evidence synthesis on-the-fly during direct patient care	• Identify sources of best evidence efficiently during direct patient care • Defend the use of a paper as best evidence for a specific patient • Accurately identify sources of bias and their impact on studies' conclusions • Calculate summary measures for a specific patient's baseline risk • Present evidence to a patient and check for understanding

Block or semester	Novice (MS, PGY-1)	• Introduce the principles of critical appraisal of the literature • Role model effective literature search skills • Review sources of bias through examples • Clarify levels of the evidence hierarchy • Introduce the skill of succinct article presentation	• Articulate a well-structured clinical question • Choose the best study design for their clinical question • Calculate likelihood ratios and correctly use a nomogram • Identify sources of bias in various studies and describe the direction of their impact • Appropriately interpret results expressed as likelihood ratios, relative risks, odds ratios, risk reductions, and number needed to treat • Accurately interpret confidence intervals • Critically appraise various study types • Apply the results of a study of therapy to an individual patient
	Inter-mediate (PGY-2)	• Teach the knowledge and skills of critical appraisal of the literature • Refine skills of electronic searching of the literature • Describe the process of establishing a diagnosis • Improve ability to detect and assess the impact of bias on study conclusions • Identify features of best published research evidence • Improve skills related to presentation of articles	• Articulate focused clinical questions • Identify high-quality papers via electronic search methods • Identify strategies for testing clinical hypotheses • List and define key critical appraisal criteria for major study types • Accurately identify bias and calibrate its impact on published studies • Appropriately interpret results expressed as likelihood ratios, relative risks, odds ratios, hazard ratios, and number needed to treat • Assess the validity of a subgroup analysis • Calculate number needed to treat for an individual patient using available relative risk data • Succinctly present an article and apply results to a clinical case
	Advanced (PGY-3, fellow, faculty)	• Teach learners to teach EBM concepts to medical students and interns	• Plan, prepare, and execute a teaching session involving one EBM concept, using clinical examples (builds on above objectives)

Classic EBM Domains and Content Areas

A curriculum in EBM can cover any or all of the following skill domains and classic content areas. Consider what your learners will need and write it out as a part of your plan ahead of time. Common examples include:

Domains [9]:

- "Doing"
  - Asking a clinical question.
  - Acquiring evidence - Searching the medical literature.
  - Appraising evidence critically.
  - Accurate interpretation of study results.
  - Applying results to patient care.
- "Using"
  - Employing pre-appraised sources of evidence to guide patient care.
- "Replicating"
  - Following the evidence based recommendations of mentors and trusted sources.
- "Communicating"
  - Communicating evidence to patients.
  - Communicating evidence to colleagues.

Content Areas:

- Searching the medical literature.
- Diagnostic testing.
- Screening.
- Therapy.
- Non-inferiority study designs.
- Harm or Causation.
- Measures of association, basic statistics, confidence intervals.
- Prognosis.
- Meta-analysis and Systematic reviews.
- Decision analysis.
- Cost-effectiveness analysis.

EBM Curriculum Methods

Many curricula will employ a mixture of different methods to conduct the teaching. While one literature review has suggested that clinically based formats demonstrate better improvement in outcomes regarding knowledge and skills, little data exists to directly compare methods. Table 1.2 lists the pros and cons of commonly used formats:

Table 1.2 Sample curricular methods

Format	Pros	Cons
Didactic	• Concise • Efficient • Address larger groups • Prepared in advance	• Passive learning • Difficult to assess learners' needs and responses
Journal Club	• Use of clinical example • Critical appraisal focus • Established in many programs	• Non-presenting learners may be passive • Informal, may not convey core concepts
Small group interactive/ workshops	• Learner involvement • Stimulate discussion • Flexibility, change direction as needed • Experiential	• Address smaller groups • Requires more faculty time • Impact of learner level may create variability
Clinical (bedside or on rounds, inpatient or outpatient)	• Grounding in clinical context may lead to deeper learning and retention • Role model real-time use of resources	• Difficult to incorporate into the pace of clinical work • Faculty readiness and availability
Web based	• Prepare in advance • No faculty time needed for teaching • Wide range of options for content and formats, can be experiential	• May be difficult to assess learners' needs and provide feedback • May lack direct clinical relevance

Selecting Good Teaching Papers

No matter the format you select, many EBM curricula involve selecting articles to illustrate teaching points. This is a critical step! Putting thought in ahead of time will likely reap rewards in terms of the engagement of learners and the impact of the curriculum. We recommend keeping the following factors in mind as you select teaching articles:

- Timely—adds value as a clinical pearl in addition to the EBM pearl; high yield for learners.
- Teaching points—the article must illustrate the teaching point you are driving at. If you want learners to calculate absolute and relative risk reductions, for instance, make sure it is an article where the event rates are easy to find and mathematically manageable. The same idea applies to any of the multitude of potential teaching points.
- "Totality"—The totality of the papers chosen across a curriculum should represent a wide variety of article types and article quality. Avoid choosing only flawed papers, or only strong papers! Aim for a mix of both.

In addition, it is important to remember that while you may sometimes utilize an entire paper, it is not required! You may want to extract key paragraphs or figures to illustrate your teaching point, and only provide those. If you are teaching from an entire paper, it helps to have learners read it ahead of time and prepare for the session, unless you will provide time to read it in the session. Another approach to using a full paper in a teaching setting is to "pre-digest" it—mark it up with labels and highlights to allow learners to get to the important areas faster. How much of the article you decide to employ will vary with your time available, your teaching format, and learning objectives.

Putting it All Together

Now, we suggest you put all of these factors together into an EBM Curricular Proposal. This proposal can function as a starting point for discussion with stakeholders in your environment as you "make the case" for your curriculum. See Table 1.3 for a summary.

Table 1.3 EBM Curriculum Planning Worksheet

Learners	
Setting	
Time Frame	
Goals	
Objectives	
Content	
Methods	
Support/ Stakeholders	

References

1. Sackett DL, Rosenberg WMC, et al. Evidence based medicine: what it is and what it isn't. BMJ. 1996;312:71–2.
2. Haynes RB, Sackett DL, Guyatt GH, Tugwell P. Clinical epidemiology: how to do clinical practice research. 3rd ed. Lipincott Williams and Wilkins; 2005.
3. Guyatt GH. Evidence-based medicine. ACP J Club. 1991;114:A16.
4. Guyatt G, Rennie D, Meade MO, Cook DJ. Users' guides to the medical literature: a manual for evidence-based clinical practice. 3rd ed. Chicago: American Medical Association; 2015.
5. Burke AE, Benson B, et al. Domain of competence: practice based learning and improvement. Acad Pediatr. 2014;14:S38–54.
6. LCME Functions and structure of a medical school: standards for accreditation of medical education programs leading to the MD degree. March 2018, Association of American Medical Colleges and American Medical Association.
7. Diamond R. Designing and assessing courses & curricula: a practical guide. 3rd ed. San Francisco: Jossey-Bass; 1998.
8. Bloom B, editor. Taxonomy of educational objectives: the classification of educational goals. Handbook 1: cognitive domain. New York: David McKay; 1956.
9. Straus SE, Green ML, Bell DS, et al. For the SGIM evidence-based medicine task force. Evaluating the teaching of evidence-based medicine: conceptual framework. BMJ. 2004;329:1029.

Clinical Question and Study Design

2

Daniella A. Zipkin and Deepa Rani Nandiwada

Guide for the Teacher

Introducing learners to the practice of evidence-based medicine should begin with an understanding of the importance of applying evidence-based medicine (EBM) in everyday clinical decision making and the rapid evolution of clinical practice and guidelines. We recommend covering the following three foundational topics up front: (1) asking a clinical question, (2) selecting a study design which answers your question, and (3) the concepts of bias and random error.

Starting with how to ask a clinical question frames all of EBM where it truly belongs—squarely with the patient. Learners may have been exposed to journal club settings which are common, and often focus on pulling up a big paper and appraising it, without mention of a patient. We recommend steering learners away from this, as there is significant evidence that real-time evidence-based learning (in the clinics, on rounds, or with patient cases) is more effective

Supplementary Information The online version contains supplementary material available at [https://doi.org/10.1007/978-3-031-11174-7_2].

D. A. Zipkin (✉)
Department of Medicine, Duke University Health System,
Duke University School of Medicine, Durham, NC, USA
e-mail: daniella.zipkin@duke.edu

D. R. Nandiwada
Division of General Internal Medicine, Department of Medicine, Penn Center for Primary Care Penn Presbyterian Hospital, University of Pennsylvania Perelman School of Medicine, Philadelphia, PA, USA
e-mail: deepa.nandiwada@pennmedicine.upenn.edu

D. A. Zipkin (ed.), *Teaching Evidence-Based Medicine*,
https://doi.org/10.1007/978-3-031-11174-7_2

than journal clubs and group didactics alone, since the latter create a temporal and physical space between the evidence and the patient (1–6). Because we can't possibly function as giant repositories of information and we are unlikely to store all of the journal club discussions we have heard in a way that allows those articles to be useful to us later, we should start with an actual patient question and ground our teaching in the process of gathering and assessing evidence to answer it. The medical literature is dynamic, not static, and looking up the same question over the years is not redundant. Instead it will result in new answers as the evidence evolves, ensuring that learners are on top of the latest developments. Just as clinical medicine begins with a good history and physical exam, so should exploring evidence begin with a good question.

Moving on to study design ensures that learners approach the remainder of the material with some key terminology and an understanding of the pros and cons of various designs to be able to critically assess the literature.

Finally, we have found that rounding out the introductory session with a conversation about bias and random error provides learners with a framework for assessing the impact of any one study in the sea of all that is known or not known about a topic. *Bias* is analogous to anything that compromises *accuracy* of a study, and *random error* is analogous to lack of *precision*. These concepts are the two primary ways in which we may deviate from the truth, and presenting them with some high yield visual aids in the beginning of an EBM curriculum reaps many rewards in explaining things that arise in future sessions.

Curriculum Development

Before launching any EBM teaching plan, spend some time thinking through your context and your plan.

What resources are already available at your institution?
Who are your learners? What is their level of understanding of the material? What do they need from the teaching? What are their goals?
When will the sessions occur? Will clinical duties conflict with participation?
What is your time frame, and how will teaching time be distributed?
Who are the faculty? What is their level of experience with the content and with teaching in general?
Who are the stakeholders to whom you will be accountable?
Will teaching sessions be linked, building on each other, or will they stand alone?
Can learners be expected to do preparatory work before their sessions, or follow-up work after?
How will you assess the learners' uptake of the curriculum, in terms of knowledge, attitudes, and behaviors?

Lay out your teaching plan in advance, and then utilize this book in adapting the curricular pieces to your local environment. Teaching tips are all accompanied by the time you might expect them to take.

Teaching Methods:

Consider employing the following principles in your teaching plans:

State objectives for each session utilizing language of measurable behaviors – what will the learner be able to DO after the session?
Engage the learner through interaction from the beginning by utilizing clinical cases.
Avoid "lectures"; Be a facilitator – the best gauge of a successful teaching session is when the learners speak more than the teacher!
Provide tools they can work with that help them see the material from more than one vantage point.
Repeat information in auditory and visual formats.
Engage learners by having them work through questions or solve problems independently or in small groups.
Conclude with take home points, key pearls to remember.

Introduction to Evidence Based Medicine:

The Evidence Cycle, and Asking a Clinical Question

Objectives

By the end of this session, learners will be able to

1. Define the components of a well-formed clinical question.
2. Formulate their own clinical question.
3. Decide which type of question they are asking and which type of study is most suitable to answer it.

Evidence based medicine begins and ends with the patient. Patient stories make up the foundation of what we do in medicine. The ways in which we guide and help patients are formed from our schooling, our clinical experience, and our ability to ask new questions and incorporate the answers into opportunities for shared clinical decision making. Keeping the key steps outlined in Fig. 2.1 in mind helps to move through a process that can otherwise feel overwhelming due to the sheer volume of potential sources of answers. It is also vital to acknowledge that we are not experts in all aspects of medicine and that this cycle will be used throughout a physician's

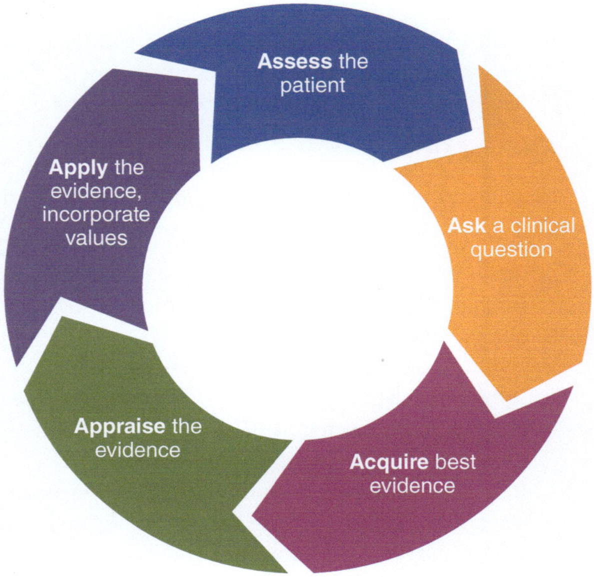

Fig. 2.1 The Evidence Cycle. EBM begins with assessing the patient, then moves to asking a question, acquiring best evidence, appraising the evidence, and applying that evidence back to the patient while incorporating patient values

entire career. Answers to clinical questions are readily available, and the better we frame our clinical question, the more likely we are to find the right answer. The components of your question are the terms you will use in your Medline search to find the most fitting answer. This session is aimed at outlining your question in the optimal format in order to facilitate your literature search.

Anatomy of a Question

It is essential to be explicit about what you are asking when posing a question about a patient. Questions come in two general flavors: *background* questions and *foreground* questions. Background questions are more general, often related to pathophysiology, epidemiology, or the natural history of disease. Foreground questions are more granular and refer to a particular feature of the condition in question, such as how best to make the diagnosis, how to treat it, or what to expect prognostically based on factors the patient possesses. Background questions may be "what is that?", while foreground questions may ask "what is the most effective intervention for that?". As the level of expertise on a topic develops, questions tend to evolve from background to foreground questions. The format listed in the Box is best suited for foreground questions, but can be adapted to background questions as well – sometimes by leaving out the intervention and/or control (Box 2.1).

Box 2.1 Components of the Clinical Question
P = *Population* (Which patients or problem? Be specific!)
I = *Intervention* (or *exposure* or *test* or *prognostic* factor).
C = *Control or comparison* (if appropriate).
O = *Outcomes* (What is the clinical goal?)

Let us practice setting up a few questions. Specify each component of the question based upon the clinical scenario. For example:

- Not enough info: "what is the best treatment for GERD?"
- Better: "are proton pump inhibitors more effective than H2 blockers for the alleviation of GERD symptoms in adults who do not have peptic ulcer disease?"
  - P = adults with Dx of GERD, no PUD
  - I = PPI
  - C = H2 blockers
  - O = symptom relief.

For the following examples, formulate the PICO for each question:

- Not enough info: "should this patient with recent MI take Ezetemibe?"
- Better: "should this woman with MI in the preceding thirty days take Ezetemibe with her statin in order to further reduce cardiovascular events?"
  - P =
  - I =
  - C =
  - O =
- Try this one: "Does a high fat diet cause breast cancer in women over 40?" (an exposure, not an intervention).
  - P =
  - I =
  - C =
  - O =

Deciding on the Type of Question

As you think of your question, you will first decide upon the patient population, the intervention or exposure, the control, and the outcome of interest. However, a crucial part to finding the answer is considering what type of question you are asking. Is it a question of the best diagnostic test to order, the prevalence of disease, the prognosis, or therapy? Are there different ways to approach the question? For example, sometimes we want to know the accuracy of a diagnostic test, which is observational, but sometimes we want to know the benefits of applying that diagnostic test in a clinical algorithm, which is an intervention. The next question to ask is, "what is the optimal study design for answering this question?" This will allow you to critically appraise the evidence to ensure your answer meets quality standards. *We will sort through study designs to match your questions in the next section.*

Where to Find Answers

Medical Databases can be a good source for general topic reviews and *background questions*. Some databases are based on a substantial amount of expert opinion – wording such as "our practice is to…" may indicate this. Look for systematically researched comprehensive resources for clinical decision making, where references to all source data are available, and the quality of the evidence is rated. These resources can be highly valuable as a first step, but it is vital that you look at the references to ensure the information provided is targeted at the patient you are caring for.

Individual studies make up the focus of the rest of this course. We will discuss how to find what you need on *PubMed*, the National Library of Medicine's primary database for published medical research. Figure 2.2 illustrates how various study types get closer to approximating the truth.

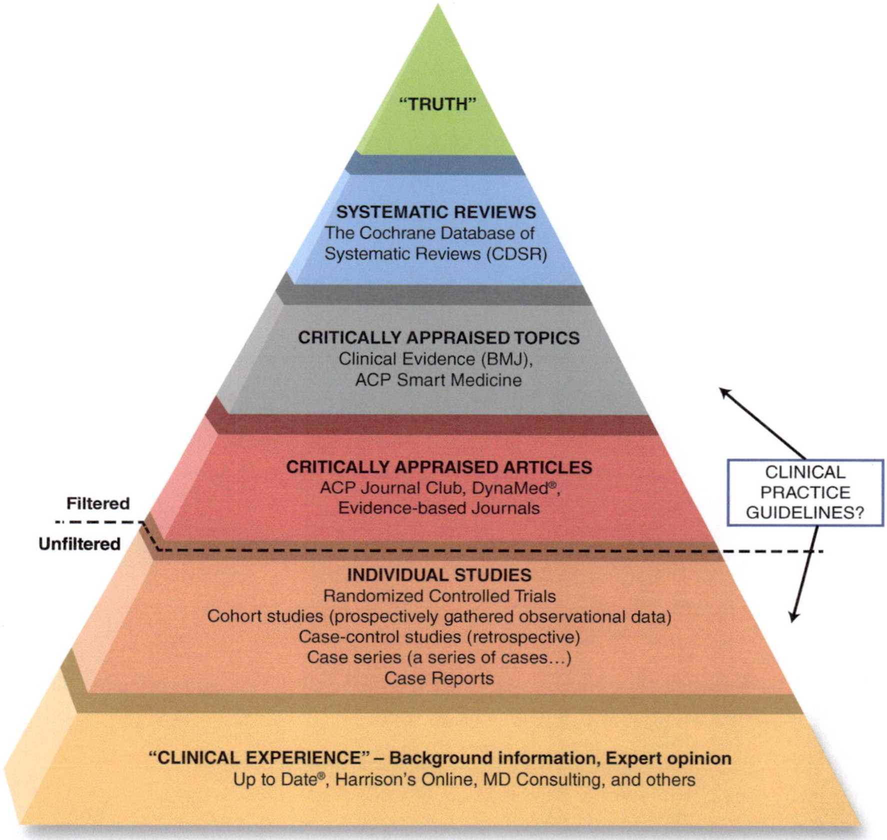

Fig. 2.2 The Hierarchy of Evidence. The truth is what we are searching for. This pyramid diagram illustrates how close to the truth different sources of evidence can get, when conducted well. "Filtered" sources are those that utilize a stated methodology to select and combine pieces of evidence, and all should include a system of assessing the level of bias in those sources. Individual studies in the medical literature are unfiltered, and EBM courses are designed to give readers the skills to appraise them independently. Note that clinical practice guidelines will vary by guiding organization, and that organization's decisions regarding which evidence to incorporate and how rigorously to grade the level of bias in the evidence sources

TEACH IT!!

Asking a Clinical Question

10 min:

Prepare the learners ahead of time—let them know they will be asking their own clinical questions and they should think about questions that have arisen recently in the context of patient care. For early medical students you can prepare a brief clinical vignette ahead of time.

Write "P" "I" "C" "O" on the board and ask the group for an example of a question.

When someone states a question, start filling in the PICO items from their question, asking for clarification when needed.

If they have shared a background question, point out how the "intervention" and "control" categories are not necessarily applicable. Re-write a related PICO on a potential therapy question about the same condition. Point out the differences, and mention that it's important to clarify for yourself what angle you're taking on the question because it will inform how you search the literature later.

If they start with a therapy question, do the same thing in reverse: re-write a related PICO on the corresponding background question, and point out how they differ.

Take at least one more learner's question, and demonstrate the same principle, this time asking the group to fill in the categories.

Have every learner write out their PICO questions on a piece of paper or worksheet, adding the type of question and the type of study they will look for.

Study Design

Objectives

By the end of this session, learners will be able to

1. Describe the design features of the major study types,
2. Identify which type of study design is best suited to answer different types of questions,
3. Define the concepts of bias and random error.

Here we review different sorts of studies, with their common uses, and mention of some of their drawbacks. We start with a table matching up types of questions with the studies we find to answer them in Table 2.1. See the paragraphs which follow for more explanations, including the types of bias found in each study design.

Table 2.1 Study designs which address different types of clinical questions

Type of question	Possible study designs
Diagnostic testing	Cross-sectional, cohort
Therapy or prevention	RCT
Screening	RCT (screening is an intervention, too!)
Causation or harm	RCT > cohort > case control > case series
Prognosis	Cohort > case series
Natural history	Cohort > case series
Prevalence	Cross-sectional
Incidence	Cohort

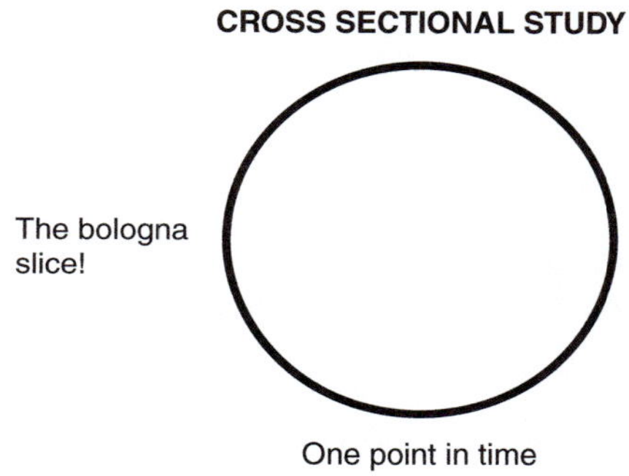

Fig. 2.3 Cross-sectional Study

Case Series

Design: A description of a series of subjects with a similar diagnosis.

Types of Questions Answered: Descriptive and observational questions, such as those involving the natural history of disease, can be addressed. Signs and symptoms associated with various disease outcomes can be described. While case series are typically more than one case, individual case reports can be helpful in describing rare disease processes. The validity of these studies hinges on the population sampled, and its relevance to your population of interest. These studies are *launching points* for further hypothesis testing about these populations.

Cross-Sectional Studies

Design: A population sample where each participant contributes measurements on a single occasion, as shown in Fig. 2.3.

Types of questions answered: Examining networks of causal links, and determining *prevalence*. Generally descriptive, cross-sectional studies cannot establish cause and effect. Most diagnostic testing studies are cross-sectional, in that a diagnostic test is performed on the entire group of subjects, and then the test of interest is compared to the results of the gold standard. The "single point in time" for each subject should occur close enough in time to be measuring the same thing for each subject. It need not be on the same actual day. These subjects are not followed forward prospectively.

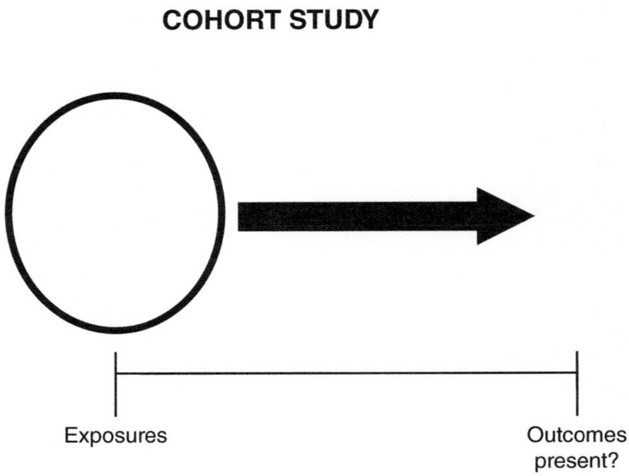

Fig. 2.4 Cohort Study

Cohort Studies

Design: Observational studies which follow groups of subjects over time, longitudinally, as shown in Fig. 2.4.

Prospective—Define the sample of patients and measure predictors or exposures, then follow forward for outcomes.
Retrospective—Typically, retrospective cohort refers to a *retrospective* analysis of previously gathered *prospective* data. This is useful when new questions arise at the end of a cohort study which can be answered with the data already gathered. Data has still been gathered *prospectively*.
The difference between prospective and retrospective cohorts is the position of the investigator. The investigator sits at the beginning of the study in a prospective design, and asks a question after the study in a retrospective design.

Types of Questions Answered: Describe the *incidence* or natural history of certain conditions over time, analyze associations between exposures and outcomes, or evaluate a diagnostic test.

Case-Control Studies

Design: Retrospective analysis of one group of subjects with a known disease and one without it (control group), looking backward in time to find differences in predictors, via patient interview or chart review or stored samples, as shown in Fig. 2.5.

Variation: Nested Case-control—Perform the retrospective analysis within a cohort previously followed. Identify cases within a cohort study who developed an outcome, and controls who did not, and then retrieve predictor variable data already collected. This can be more reliable if the data was collected well initially.

Fig. 2.5 Case Control Study

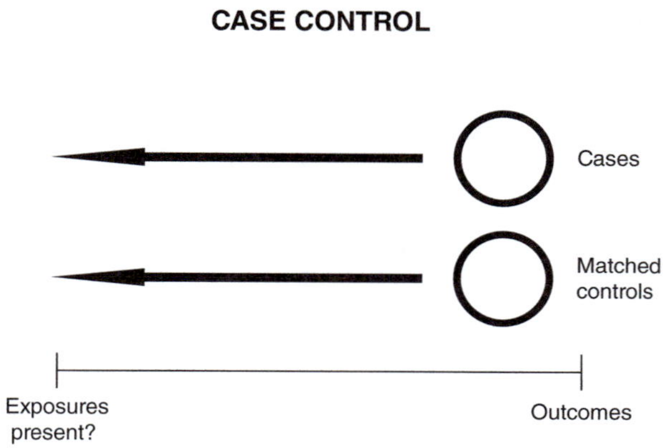

Types of questions answered: Useful for *rare* diseases due to the high yield of information from relatively few subjects, but susceptible to bias and not useful to establish incidence or prevalence. Cases identified may not be representative of all cases with the disease due to lack of presenting to medical attention, misdiagnosis, or death before diagnosis.

All of the designs above are still observational. We have not yet intervened or performed an experiment.... now, we look at interventions:

Clinical Trials (Gold Standard: Randomized Controlled Trials)

Design: An intervention or treatment is given, groups are allocated to different treatments, and outcomes are observed, as shown in Fig. 2.6. Key elements include entry criteria, sample size, randomization, blinding, controls, and choice of outcomes measured.

Types of questions answered: Randomized controlled trials are the best study design for questions of causality, screening, treatment, prevention, and harm. By comparing two groups that are treated equally in all respects except for the intervention or variable of interest, it is reasonable to attribute differences in outcomes to that intervention or variable.

Review: A non-systematic review of the literature on a particular topic. Articles selected for the review are at the discretion of the authors.

Systematic Review: A methodologically systematic, rigorous approach to collecting all studies in the literature which answer a particular clinical question. In a systematic review, the studies themselves are the "subjects," complete with inclusion and exclusion criteria. See the chapter on Systematic Reviews for more detail.

Meta-analysis: A study which calculates summary effect sizes for a group of studies. Meta-analysis may be performed on systematically reviewed studies. Many systematic reviews also perform meta-analyses on the study outcomes, however, some remain descriptive when the outcomes cannot be mathematically combined.

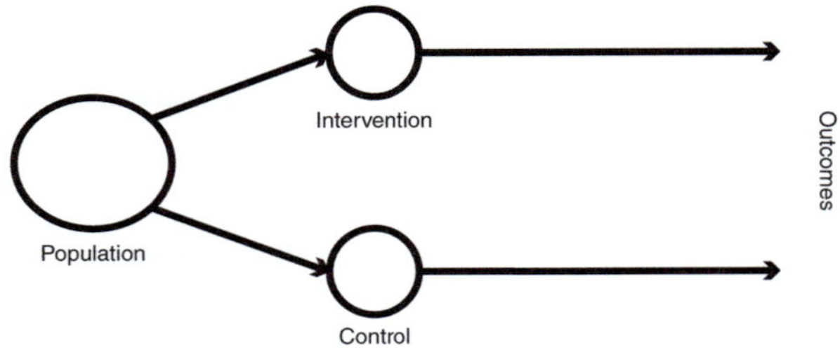

Fig. 2.6 Randomized Controlled Trial

TEACH IT!!

Study Design

15–30 min:

Tell the group you are going to share some scenarios, and you want them to tell you the study design. Here we will share a clinical example we use which can illustrate some of these concepts succinctly. This also blends with the clinical scenario we use in the Harm section, and can be a lead-in to that discussion.

Scenario 1: Draw a circle on the board. You are doing a survey study of college kids by setting up a table on the quad for 3 months of the year and asking for volunteers to take your survey as they walk by. Your survey asks about medical history, diet, exercise, tobacco, alcohol, drug use, and sexual history. You ask them to fill it out only once. At the end of the study, you publish a paper describing the health habits of college kids today.

Answer: Cross-sectional. Everyone contributes data at one point in time. These studies provide information on prevalence.

Scenario 2: You are able to enroll all of the students who take your survey for longer term follow-up. You intend to repeat the survey every 2 years for the next 20 years. You will remove their identifying information from the data.

Answer: Cohort study. Draw a horizontal line moving forward from the circle you drew, with a hash mark at the end of the line. Label the circle "exposures" and the hash mark "outcomes." These studies provide information on incidence.

Share a real life example: Imagine diet soda consumption was found to be associated with diabetes. (This real example is discussed in more detail in Chap. 6: Harm and Causation).

Add a discussion of prospective cohort vs retrospective cohort. In a contrasting color, draw a stick figure above the exposures circle at the beginning, and another stick figure after the outcomes. Point out that the cohort is always conducted moving forward in prospective fashion. The only that changes in retrospective cohorts is the vantage point of the investigator. Investigators may go back to previously conducted cohorts and ask a new question. This is legitimate, and encouraged! Cohort designers know they are creating a data source others will use. Advantages include the lower cost and less time needed to conduct the study. Disadvantages are that you are limited to which data was collected, and how it was collected, at the beginning of the cohort.

Scenario 3: Tell the group you are very interested in further exploring this diet soda/diabetes connection, but you have a limited budget. You will gather a group of patients with diabetes, and a group of patients without diabetes, and then ask them about their history of diet soda consumption.

Answer: Case Control. Draw two squares on the right hand side of the board. Draw horizontal lines coming from the squares and moving left, backwards in time. Put hash marks at the left end of the lines. Label the squares "outcome," and the hash marks "exposure."

Discuss how the case control study was built. How were the patients selected, and where were they recruited? Newspaper ads? Primary care offices? Endocrinology offices? Each of these decisions changes the nature of the population you will recruit, and the subsequent findings. Controls are often recruited via some matching regarding age, gender, and socioeconomic status. Is this sufficient? What would happen if you oversampled for obese patients among the controls? You'd be making the controls more similar to the cases. Would this make it easier, or harder, to find differences in the exposure? Harder! Notice that building a more "rigorous" comparator group, as similar as possible to the cases with the exception of the condition of interest, makes it harder to find differences in exposure and is not in the interests of the investigators.

Discuss the process of looking back to find out about exposures and address possible sources of bias. Asking patients is fraught with recall bias and social appropriateness biases (patients telling investigators what they think they want to hear). Can we use the medical record? This data was not likely to have been captured. Looking back is challenging, and never a perfect process.

Because of all of these biases, case control studies should be limited to times when the condition is RARE, or when the outcome is a harm that cannot be studied prospectively for ethical reasons. Diabetes is not rare, and should really never be studied in this way. Case control studies also offer the advantage of being less costly and taking less time than prospective studies, so we will see them often when budgets and time are tight. Because of their limitations, they should be considered hypothesis generating, and confirmed by prospective studies whenever possible.

Scenario 4: Tell the group you are still worried about this connection between diet soda and diabetes, so you're going to design an experiment where you assign half of your subjects to receive only diet soda and half of your subjects to receive a comparator beverage, then follow them forward to look for incident diabetes.

Answer: Randomized Controlled Trial.

This is a great time to talk about a topic often left out of the conversation of risk of bias: the *choice of comparator*. Ask the group, what should the comparator beverage be? Often they will answer "water" or "nothing" or "regular soda." Pause for a moment. Point out that, to some degree, the choice of comparator depends on who we are and what we hope to find. If we believe that there is something inherently wrong with diet soda and it's bad for you, we will likely choose water or nothing. If we are sponsored by the diet soda makers, and we live in a fictional world where diet soda and regular soda are made by different companies, we would likely choose regular soda as the comparator, to put our product in the best light possible. This dilemma of bias imparted by how we choose the comparator is real, and happens in the literature. It is not uncommon for investigators to stack the deck in favor of the finding they want.

Optional: Continue the conversation by reviewing the more common areas for bias in RCTs and how RCTs try to combat them, via randomization, allocation concealment, equal treatment, blinding, completeness of follow-up, and intention to treat. With each one, ask the group why it's important, how to do it well, and how it spreads the confounding more evenly across the groups and keeps all things equal other than the intervention of interest. These topics are covered in detail in the chapter on Therapy.

30 min:

For learners who benefit from individual reading and written work, consider preparing a worksheet with scenarios similar to those above ahead of time. Have learners read the scenarios and fill in a table of study design, with the following features:

Types of questions answered.

Time horizon—prospective or retrospective.

Gathering subjects at time of exposure vs outcome.

Sources of bias.

Pros and cons.

60 min:

If you have more time, or a larger group, make it interactive!

Gather volunteers to help you. Prepare cards ahead of time for them to hold, labeled "exposure," "outcome," and "time" or a clock. Use a ball (or other relatively safe object) and have the "exposure" volunteer and the "outcome" volunteer throw the ball in the direction of inquiry, demonstrating cohorts and case controls, as well as randomized controlled trials. Make the point that randomized trials are also moving from exposures to outcomes – they are just a variant of cohorts which add randomized groups assigned to the exposure.

Bias and Random Error

Bias leads to outcomes which are *systematic* deviations from the truth. Simply stated, bias is anything that takes us further from the truth. The deviation has a *direction*, it can serve to either underestimate or overestimate the underlying benefit or harm of an intervention. Bias will be present if treatment and control patients differ in substantial ways at the start of the study, or if they are treated differently during the course of the study, or if outcomes are measured differently between groups. Bias generally arises from flaws in study design. Several examples of biases were mentioned in the context of the study designs above.

As we critically appraise the risk of bias of various studies throughout this book, we are looking for features in those study designs that minimize bias. Any time you identify an issue within a study that causes bias, decide for yourself in which direction the bias might go, and decide if that has an important impact on your interpretation of the study.

Random error reflects the fact that any one measurement has some degree of error built in. If we repeat a study multiple times, we will get many estimates of the truth. The more times we repeat a study, or the greater the number of subjects in a study, the tighter will be the distribution of results around the truth. In other words, *increasing the number of participants in the study or the number of outcome observations that participants have will REDUCE random error*. We will soon see that this is reflected in the confidence interval. If you see a well designed study arrive at a result with a wide confidence interval, you should ask yourself, was the sample size or the number of outcome event too small?

Imagine a coin flip. You know that there is a 50% chance of either heads or tails. In this case, 50% is the "truth." If you flip a coin ten times, you may easily have seven heads and three tails. If you flip it 100 times, you may have 65 heads and 35 tails. If you flip it 1000 times, or 10,000 times, you will expect to get closer and closer to 50%.

To minimize *bias*, a study must be well designed and well executed. To minimize *random error*, a study must be large, or must be repeated and confirmed.

In studies of therapeutics, randomized controlled designs minimize bias when they are well done. Observational designs such as cohort studies are vulnerable to more bias, often in the form of confounding.

Imagine that the large circle in the center represents the "truth" (keeping in mind that in reality, we never know exactly where the truth lies). The smaller dots represent the point estimates from hypothetical individual studies, if repeated multiple times. We can use the example of a therapy question, where a well done randomized trial would be our optimal study design. In scenario A, we have little bias, as the point estimates are centered evenly about the truth, and we have little random error, as the spread of potential results around the truth is minimal. This could represent large (little random error) RCTs (little bias). In scenario B, we have little bias, as the point estimates are still centered evenly about the truth, but we see more random error, as the spread is wider. This could represent small RCTs. In scenario C, we have a lot of bias, as we are nowhere near the truth, but very little random error (in other words, we are wrong, but we don't know it, and we may feel very sure of ourselves!). In this figure, we represent bias as "fan," blowing us off the truth—since bias is systematic error and has a direction to it. This could represent a large (little random error) cohort study (biased by confounding variables). Finally, in scenario D we see the worst of both worlds, a lot of bias, and a lot of random error, as may be found in a small cohort study for a question of therapy.

One of the most well known examples of bias due to study design involves post-menopausal hormone replacement therapy. Cohort studies published in the 1990s suggested a reduction in cardiovascular disease with HRT, but randomized trials published beginning in 2002 found lack of benefit, and even slight harm with HRT. Why did the cohort studies originally report benefit? Confounding variables, or other variables related to women choosing to take HRT, were at play – those women were healthier, and likely saw their doctors more often.

Why is it important to frame these concepts of bias and random error? Many studies we encounter on therapy questions, for instance, tend to be small, because larger trials are more challenging and require much larger budgets. They fall into scenario B. Imagine one small study – we can't know which "dot" it represents in scenario B, but let us imagine for a moment that it is an outlying dot. If the study has zero bias, then it is likely that the truth will still fall into the confidence interval for that study's primary result. It may be a wide confidence interval, but the truth is in there somewhere. Now, imagine that there is not zero bias – for smaller studies, even a small amount of bias may be sufficient to move the dot off the truth, such that the confidence interval may no longer include the truth. This is how low numbers leading to a lot of random error and a small amount of bias may conspire to make the results of small studies inaccurate, even when the p-value is statistically significant!! P-values do not protect us from this phenomenon.

TEACH IT!!

Bias and Random Error

While not all courses in evidence-based medicine take time to review bias and random error as a unique topic, we believe it is foundational content which helps learners understand issues in all of the other teaching modules in this book.

15–30 min:

This teaching technique described here is also discussed in Video 2.1 which accompanies this chapter.

Draw Fig. 2.7 on the board or create it as a slide or worksheet for learners to use in this session.

Ask the group to define "bias." Wait for responses. They will generally move to some version of "takes you away from the truth." Ask them if it has a direction away from the truth? The answer is yes, though you may not always know the direction!

Now ask them to define random error. This term tends to be familiar but learners often haven't verbalized a definition. Random error is the inherent error in any measurement, and has no particular direction. Random error is best illustrated with a coin flip visualization. Ask the group to imagine you have a coin in your hand—the "truth" is that there is a 50% probability of heads showing up. If you flip the coin 10 times, will you get 5 heads and 5 tails? Likely not! If you flip 100 times, will you get 50 and 50? Probably not, but you'll get closer. How about 1000 times? 10,000 times? You can imagine the precision of our estimate improves with the increasing number of observations. This reduces the random error. Large sample sizes and large numbers of outcome events reduce random error—and in the literature, we see this in the tighter confidence intervals.

Now that you have defined bias and random error, look at the scenarios on the board. Ask the group to rate the bias and random error of each scenario, in turn, pausing with each one. Put labels beneath them to rate the Bias and Random Error as low or high. You will gradually create (Fig. 2.8). Provide the equivalent study design and study size, as if it were a therapy question where RCTs would be the optimal design. Scenario #1 is both low bias and low random error. So it can represent a collection of large RCTs. Scenario #2 is low bias, but high random error, so it can represent a collection of small RCTs. Scenario #3 is high bias, but low random error. Does it represent RCTs at all? Probably not—go ahead and label it large cohorts. Notice that we can represent bias as a "fan," "blowing us off the truth." Looking again at #3, you might say that scenario is, "dead wrong, but really sure of myself!". This usually gets a laugh out of your learners, and leads to the point that the dot of "truth" in the center is something we cannot see. We are doing our best to assess how good any piece of evidence is at estimating the truth. When we cover up the dot of truth, Scenario #1 and Scenario #3 look a lot alike! Statistically significant p-values and tight confidence intervals do not tell you if the source of the data is reliable. We must be able to assess it ourselves.

You can also take this as an opportunity to look at Scenario #1 and #2 and discuss how one can become the other. How do we move from a high random error scenario to a low random error scenario? Either design a much larger study, or conduct a systematic review of multiple studies on the question and combine them in a meta-analysis. Conversely, how do we move from a low random error situation to a high random error situation? By having a high rate of loss to follow-up, a lower than expected event rate, looking at a sub-group of the study, and stopping the trial early. (See the separate discussion on teaching about trials stopped early in the Therapy chapter.) You may create something similar to Fig. 2.9.

Bias and Random Error, continued: Dealing with one small positive trial in the universe of truth

Focus for a moment on Scenario #2, a broad cloud centered on the truth. One learner once asked, "isn't the truth captured in the confidence interval?". That is a great question to review with each group when you teach this. Yes, in fact, if there is zero or minimal bias as the hypothetical diagram indicates, the truth should still be somewhere in that confidence interval. Using (Fig. 2.9), pick an outlying dot and draw a confidence interval in a contrasting color which overlaps with the central dot of truth. Explain that you can't ever know which dot you are, but let's say for a moment you are this outlying dot. If bias were truly zero, the truth is very likely to be in that confidence interval—in fact, there's a 95% chance that it is! However, if there is even a small amount of bias, represented in the figure as a "smaller" fan, it could shift to point estimate off the truth enough so that the confidence interval no longer includes the truth—even when it's "statistically significant"!! How much bias this requires, we cannot know. Where the truth really lies and whether this study is a good estimate of it is unknown. We emphasize with learners that the concept we want them to grasp is that smaller studies are more VULNERABLE to this happening, even with only a little bit of bias. Any time you see a reasonably well done RCT which is small and finds a difference, you must wonder if this bias and random error issue has shifted it off the truth. This is also the reason we need studies to be repeated, increasing our confidence in a true effect.

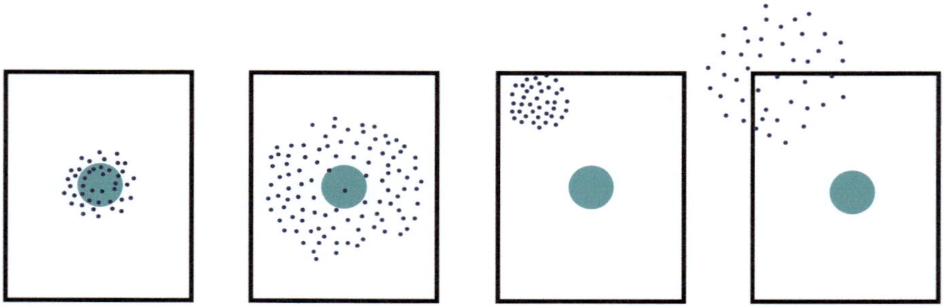

Fig. 2.7 Bias and Random Error Diagram

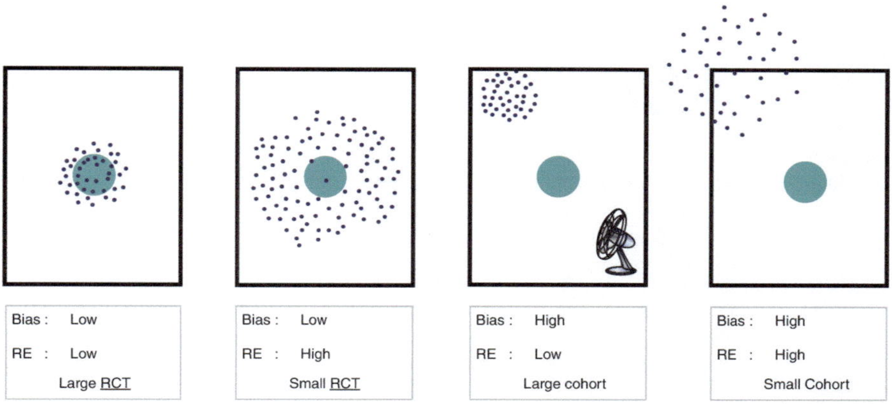

Fig. 2.8 Bias and Random Error

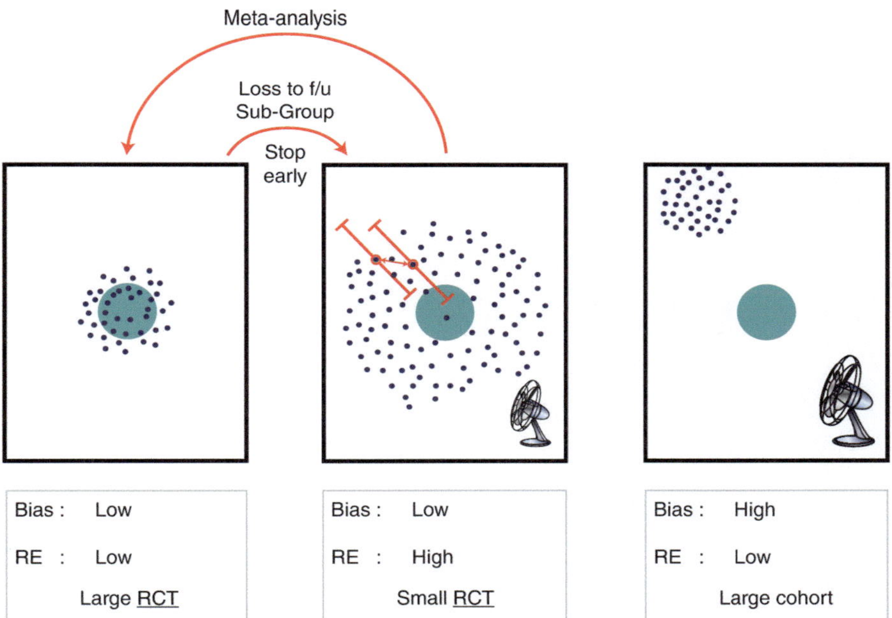

Fig. 2.9 Bias and Random Error Answers

References

1. Thom DH, et al. Description and evaluation of an EBM curriculum using a block rotation. BMC Med Educ. 2004;4:19.
2. Schilling L, Steiner J, Lundahl K, et al. Residents' patient-specific clinical questions: opportunities for evidence-based learning. Acad Med. 2005;80(1):51–6.
3. Hatala R, Keitz SA, at el. Beyond journal clubs: moving toward an integrated evidence-based medicine curriculum. J Gen Intern Med. 2006;21:538–41.
4. George P, et al. Using a learning coach to teach residents evidence-based medicine. Fam Med. 2012;44(5):351–4.
5. Swennen M, Van de Heijden G, Boeije M, et al. Doctors perceptions and use of evidence-based medicine: a systematic review and thematic synthesis of qualitative studies. Acad Med. 2013;88(9):1384–96.
6. Kenefick C, et al. Partnering with residents for evidence-based practice. Med Ref Serv Q. 2013;32(4):385–95.

Searching the Medical Literature

3

Megan von Isenburg and Daniella A. Zipkin

Guide for the teacher

This chapter focuses on the "acquire" step of the classic steps in EBM. Once the learner has framed their question, they must learn the skills of effectively searching the medical literature for the best available answer. This section should be placed near the beginning of any course in EBM, and works best when learners are actively engaged in answering their own clinical questions.

This section can be taught as a collaboration between EBM faculty and medical librarians with experience in EBM teaching. We recommend starting with introductory topics such as the 5 A's, asking a clinical question, study design, and bias and random error, and then following it with a session either in a library or with access to computers and internet, to have learners practice their own search. We prepare learners before their EBM course starts by telling them that they will need to think of a clinical question—anything relating to a patient case they have actually seen—and be ready to search on the first day of class.

M. von Isenburg
Medical Center Library, School of Medicine, Duke University, Durham, NC, USA
e-mail: megan.vonisenburg@duke.edu

D. A. Zipkin (✉)
Department of Medicine, Duke University Health System,
Duke University School of Medicine, Durham, NC, USA
e-mail: daniella.zipkin@duke.edu

D. A. Zipkin (ed.), *Teaching Evidence-Based Medicine*,
https://doi.org/10.1007/978-3-031-11174-7_3

Topic Outline

- Types of resources.
  - Pre-appraised.
    - UpToDate.
    - DynaMed.
    - Cochrane.
    - ACP Journal Club.
  - Primary.
    - PubMed/MEDLINE.
    - Other databases to find articles—Google Scholar, Web of Science, Scopus.
      - Strengths/weaknesses.
  - Evaluating apps and other new tools.
    - Currency, relevance, authority, accuracy, purpose.
    - Look for references.
    - Can always test/update with quick PubMed search to ensure seeing the newest literature.
- PubMed Core Tips.
  - PICO as search strategy.
  - Subject headings and keywords.
  - Combining terms with ANDs and ORs.
  - Narrow to the relevant study design.
  - What makes a good article.
    - Relevance, generalizability, date, journal.
- Strategies for streamlining searching for evidence.
  - Working with Results of Other Primary Sources.
  - Saving your Work in PubMed.

Introduction

Practicing evidence-based medicine requires finding evidence, which typically consists of published reports of research trials or summaries of the research literature. While a proliferation of resources, computers, smartphones, and internet access has made it increasingly easy to find *an* answer to virtually any question, finding the *best* answer to a clinical question remains a clinical skill that every provider should develop.

The “Acquire” step of the evidence cycle is often synonymous with doing a PubMed search, but there are questions and situations in which PubMed may not provide the best answer. This chapter identifies and describes various evidence-based resources, tips for getting the best out of PubMed, and criteria for evaluating new resources and apps.

Table 3.1 Resources for answering background and foreground questions

Resources for Background Questions	Resources for Foreground Questions
Online textbooks	Primary resources, such as PubMed
Aggregated e-book sites, such as Clinical Key and AccessMedicine	Pre-appraised resources, such as ACP Journal Club
UpToDate	Summary resources, such as UpToDate and Cochrane Library

For the most part, the clinical questions that are asked and answered in the EBM process are foreground questions. *Foreground questions* are patient-specific questions that refer to a particular feature of the condition in question, such as how to best make the diagnosis, how to treat it, and what to expect prognostically based on factors the patient possesses. In contrast, *background questions* refer to general knowledge, such as defining a condition and estimating its prevalence and incidence in certain populations. See Table 3.1 for a listing of resources which can be used in answering both background and foreground questions.

Types of Resources

Evidence-based resources typically fall into three categories: the primary journal literature (e.g., articles reporting results of research), pre-appraised resources, and summaries. Some models further differentiate the non-primary journal literature into summaries, syntheses, guidelines, etc., but there is significant overlap among the types of information contained within these resources. It may be more helpful for providers to learn to evaluate a resource rather than to memorize the type of resource it is.

Primary Journal Literature

The "primary journal literature" simply refers to journal articles. These may be review articles, which summarize what is known on a topic, systematic review articles, which address focused clinical questions using a specific methodology to avoid bias (see more in chapter on systematic reviews), articles reporting on the results of research, which could reflect many different kinds of study designs, and opinion pieces, such as letters to the editor or perspectives.

Journal articles can be identified in two ways:

- *Browsing*: You can browse lists of all articles in a journal or lists of new articles from a current awareness alert or email. While browsing can help maintain awareness of new discoveries in a given field or topic, it is an inefficient way to find answers to clinical questions. Nonetheless, teachers of EBM may benefit from subscribing to services that distill recent high impact research in their field, because those may become a source of teaching papers.

- *Searching*: Searching can be more efficient because it can enable discovery of a relevant article based on search keyword or phrase. There are numerous different resources that can be searched, including (Box 3.1):
  - Article databases (example: PubMed/MEDLINE, CINAHL): These resources are focused around a core set of journals that were selected for inclusion. Citation information about articles (title, authors, etc.) from those journals is included, as are subject headings that describe what the article is about. These subject headings make it easier to find articles on a topic, especially when there may be multiple ways to express a concept (e.g., heart attack, MI, myocardial infarction, etc.). Some article databases do not have subject headings (e.g., Scopus, Web of Science): These resources are focused around a core set of journals selected for inclusion. They also contain citation information, such as title, authors, and abstract. Because they do not have any subject headings, you must therefore think of synonyms for any concepts for which you are searching.

Box 3.1 Commonly-Used Primary Resources

PubMed:

PubMed primarily functions as the US National Library of Medicine's free interface to the MEDLINE database. In addition to MEDLINE citations, it notably includes citations that are still in-process, meaning they have not yet been indexed with subject headings, as well as articles from PubMed Central, an open access repository, and some online books. PubMed offers features that allow users to narrow to study design and date, which makes it very useful in EBM searches.

CINAHL:

CINAHL (Cumulative Index to Nursing and Allied Health Literature) is an article database of primarily nursing journals. It features its own robust subject headings and limits and is an essential tool for answering EBP questions in nursing and allied health fields.

Web of Science:

Web of Science is an article database chiefly known for displaying the number of times an article has been cited by other articles. This feature can help users identify articles with the most citations on a topic, though cannot tell you that the article received those citations for being good or bad. This interdisciplinary database also covers social sciences and engineering, which may be appropriate for some questions. It lacks limits for study design.

Scopus:

Scopus is similar to Web of Science but is larger. It also contains the number of times an article has been cited by other articles. It includes more international journal articles than PubMed or Web of Science, which can be useful in some questions.

Google Scholar:

Google Scholar is also a freely available article database that has some full-text searching, which means it searches the full text of some (but not all) articles. Google Scholar is interdisciplinary and includes content from conference presentations, repositories, books, and other items that are not journal articles. It can be particularly useful for finding articles on named instruments (e.g., the Beck Depression Inventory), but offers no limits for study designs. The algorithm seems to favor older review articles that have been cited frequently, articles which tend to provide poor answers to clinical questions.

Pre-appraised Resources

Pre-appraised resources are resources that offer a critical appraisal of a primary research article that has usually been published elsewhere. The depth and detail of the appraisal varies by resource, but should include the primary validity criteria for the type of study published. These resources are designed to save the reader time by highlighting important studies and providing an appraisal of the study methodology and results.

When should these resources be consulted? It may be most time-efficient for a clinician to search a pre-appraised resource when their clinical question is fairly common or if an important and well-known study has been published. Pre-appraised resources contain many fewer results than a primary resource like PubMed: while this makes them easier to search, it also makes them less likely to have answers to less common questions.

Summary Resources

Summary resources offer summaries of the evidence on specific clinical topics (Box 3.2). The methodology used to summarize can vary widely and can influence the potential for bias in the resource. For example, the Cochrane Database of Systematic Reviews offers systematic reviews on clinical questions. These reviews

Box 3.2 Commonly-Used Summary Resources

Cochrane Database of Systematic Reviews:

The Cochrane Database of Systematic Reviews is a searchable online collection of systematic reviews published by the Cochrane Collaboration, an international network of researchers using high quality methods and evidence. Cochrane Reviews are often considered the gold standard of systematic reviews and are also indexed in PubMed, meaning you can also find Cochrane Reviews through PubMed searches.

DynaMed:

DynaMed provides topic overviews on clinical conditions and drugs. Topic overviews are organized in a standard outline with links to graded, high quality evidence. DynaMed continuously monitors numerous medical journals and updates the database on an ongoing basis. DynaMed is especially useful in answering clinical questions quickly. We like using it to identify prevalence of a condition and determine the effectiveness of a treatment, and get a quick overview of the evidence on a given topic.

UpToDate:

UpToDate is a commonly-used clinical reference tool that provides background and high level evidence on numerous conditions, drugs, and other treatments. UpToDate can serve as an online textbook, a point-of-care tool, and a place to gather expert opinions and connect to articles cited within the resource.

have low potential for bias because they tightly adhere to prescribed methodologies for systematic reviews, such as comprehensive searches, strict inclusion and exclusion criteria, dual- and blind screening of abstracts, and grading the evidence (see Chap. 10 for more information on systematic reviews). On the other hand, other summary resources may allow its authors to pick the studies they want to summarize with no specified inclusion criteria or evidence grading. This can result in a summary that is, in part, expert opinion because the author can select preferred treatments, older studies, and weaker evidence.

Readers must know the method used to summarize the evidence so that they can understand the potential for bias.

When should summary resources be used? Summaries are best when there is a great deal of evidence on a topic and/or when there has been conflicting evidence. Summaries are also useful in diagnoses and treatments in which the clinician has limited experience. Additionally, summaries can be useful starting places for answering a clinical question. Some clinicians may find that it is easy to start a search in a resource like UpToDate and DynaMed, then follow links to the articles in PubMed for further reading.

Apps and Other New Tools

New tools continue to be developed for both mobile devices and the web and many of these have great potential to simplify finding, saving, and accessing the evidence. Clinicians are encouraged to explore new resources and apps to find ways to streamline evidence-based practice.

Just as we use validity criteria to evaluate studies, it is important to evaluate resources to ensure that they meet the quality standards required when using information to care for patients.

1. An easy mnemonic for evaluating resources is to put them to the CRAAP test, adapted below to include prompts relevant to EBM and medical apps: (Blakesee, Sarah (2004). "The CRAAP Test". LOEX Quarterly. 31 (3).)
   (a) C: Currency.
      - How recent is the evidence within the resource?
      - How recently was the resource itself updated?
      - What is the method used to keep the resource continuously updated?

   (b) R: Relevance.
      - Is the information relevant to the clinical question at hand?
      - Is the information relevant to the clinical environment?

   (c) A: Authority.
      - Who produced the resource?
      - Does the creator have the appropriate credentials and training to produce the resource?
      - Are there references to other information within the resource?
      - Who produced the information contained within the resource?
      - Do they have the proper credentials and training to produce that information?

   (d) A: Accuracy.
      - Is the information correct?
      - Can you validate the information with external sources?
      - How good is the evidence contained within the resource? Is it graded? With what scale?
      - Do calculations function as intended?

   (e) P: Purpose.
      - Why was the resource created?

In particular, mobile apps and free websites are easy to publish and can therefore potentially have issues with quality and reliability. To evaluate apps, use the above criteria and also consider looking at reviews on the app store or on medical app review sites iMedicalApps.com.

PubMed Core Tips, Searching PubMed Efficiently

Most clinicians have searched PubMed hundreds of times, if not more. Using the evidence in clinical care requires you to be efficient and confident that you have not missed an important study. PubMed searches often result in too few or too many results. Knowing a little about how PubMed works and following some simple tips can help avoid these frustrations. In this section, we will focus on searching in the context of patient care. Searching in the context of a systematic review is more structured and exhaustive, and is beyond the scope of this book.

To Illustrate the Following PubMed Tips, We Will Use a Case as an Example

The patient is a 65-year-old male with a long history of type 2 diabetes and obesity. Otherwise his medical history is unremarkable. He does not smoke. He had knee surgery 10 years ago but otherwise has had no other major medical problems. Over the years he has tried numerous diets and exercise programs to reduce his weight but has not been very successful. His granddaughter just started high school and he wants to see her graduate and go on to college. He understands that his diabetes puts him at a high risk for heart disease and is frustrated that he cannot lose the necessary weight. His neighbor told him about a colleague at work who had his stomach stapled and as a result not only lost over 100 lbs. but also "cured" his diabetes. He wants to know if this procedure really works.

Tip 1: Start with a Focused Clinical Question

Conducting a good search in PubMed begins before you type anything in the search box. Use PICO (see Chap. 1) to identify the primary concepts relevant to the clinical question at hand. There are many pieces of information in any clinical encounter, but searching for them all will likely lead to too few results.

For this case, our PICO would be:

- P: male, 65 years old, type 2 diabetes, obese.
- I: gastric bypass surgery.
- C: standard medical care.
- O: weight loss, remission of diabetes, mortality.

Once you have developed your PICO, think about what elements are most important. These will form the basis of your search strategy. In our example, the most important elements of the PICO are:

- P: type 2 diabetes, obesity.
- I: gastric bypass surgery.
- O: remission of diabetes.

Why didn't we include age or gender? While age and gender are a part of our PICO, we typically do not search on them because it may exclude many relevant articles that simply report on the condition and intervention. It is best to search on the main patient problem, primary intervention of interest, and possibly the outcome, then use filters for age, gender, etc. if you still have too many results.

Tip 2: Search Using a Combination of Subject Headings and Keywords

Remember that PubMed is a database that contains millions of citations and abstracts to the biomedical literature, including the MEDLINE database, articles from PubMed Central, and other materials. Most articles in PubMed are indexed using subject headings called Medical Subject Headings, or MeSH terms. These MeSH terms are standardized terms that are chosen from a list and added to all indexed articles to describe what the article is about. Thus, all articles on a given topic, regardless of the terminology the author used, should be indexed to the same MeSH term. If you search using the appropriate MeSH term, you should get all indexed articles on that topic.

A keyword is a term that appears in the title or abstract of an article. Sometimes we use keywords to search when there are no good MeSH terms for a concept or when using additional synonyms may be helpful in finding the right articles.

PubMed is designed to use MeSH terms behind the scenes. If you have searched PubMed before, you have searched using MeSH terms! PubMed automatically attempts to include MeSH terms with whatever terms you type into the PubMed search box based on an algorithm. It is important to check whether PubMed has found the correct term by looking at the *Search details* on the Advanced screen.

In our example, if we type *type 2 diabetes* into the search box, *Search details* shows that our search automatically included an appropriate MeSH term, as shown in Fig. 3.1.

What does it look like when PubMed does not find an appropriate MeSH term? Imagine if we searched for a broad term like *recovery*, as in Fig. 3.2. PubMed does not map to any MeSH terms because this is too broad a concept. When PubMed does not map to a term, *Search details* shows only the term that with [All Fields] after. This is an indication that you should choose a more specific term, or look up a relevant term in the MeSH database.

What happens if PubMed maps you to the wrong MeSH term? Imagine if we searched for articles on health care workers. Checking *Search details* shows that PubMed included a MeSH term for delivery of health care and also for manpower, as shown in Fig. 3.3. Not seeing one MeSH term for the concept is an indication that perhaps there is a better MeSH term available.

To find alternative MeSH terms when *Search details* indicates that there might be a problem with your search, go to the MeSH database. This is a module within the NCBI platform that is connected to PubMed. You can search for a term and send it

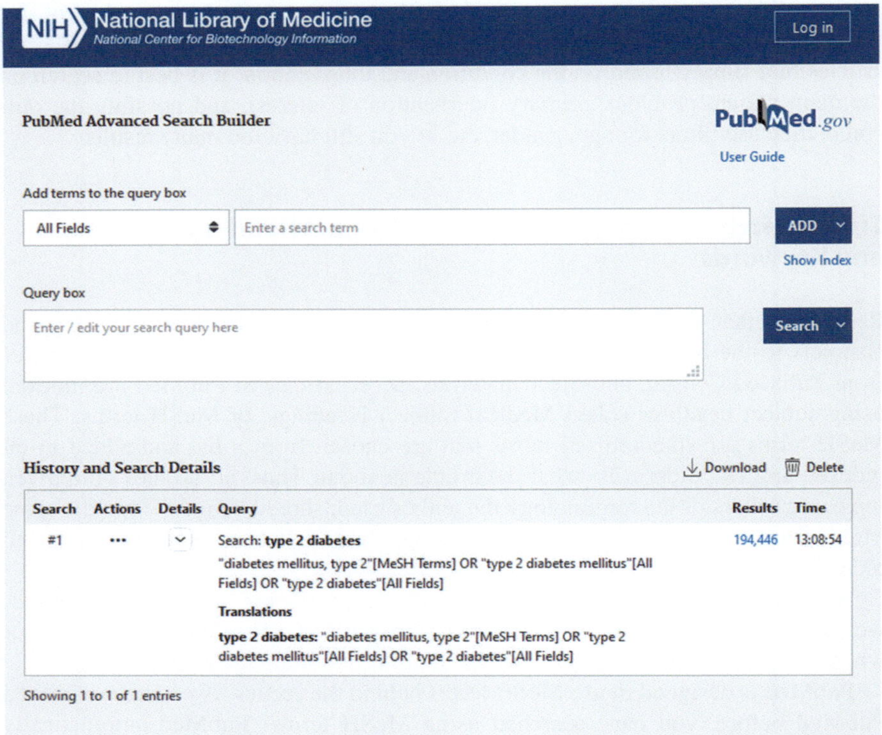

Fig. 3.1 Search Details 1

to PubMed. The steps for doing this are not complicated and may change after this book is published. At the time of publication, the steps, depicted in Fig. 3.4, are as follows:

1. Go to the MeSH database by going to the PubMed homepage and then clicking on MeSH database.
2. Type in your concept, if you have not already done so.
3. Select a MeSH term to view by clicking on the term (note: if the system only finds one MeSH term for your search term, it will appear as the only result).
4. Read the scope note to ensure it is relevant and a good match.
5. Look at the tree to see how this term fits with broader and narrower concepts.
   (a) If you search using a MeSH term, the system will also include articles indexed to narrower terms.
6. Select the term if it is appropriate and relevant.
7. Send it to PubMed.

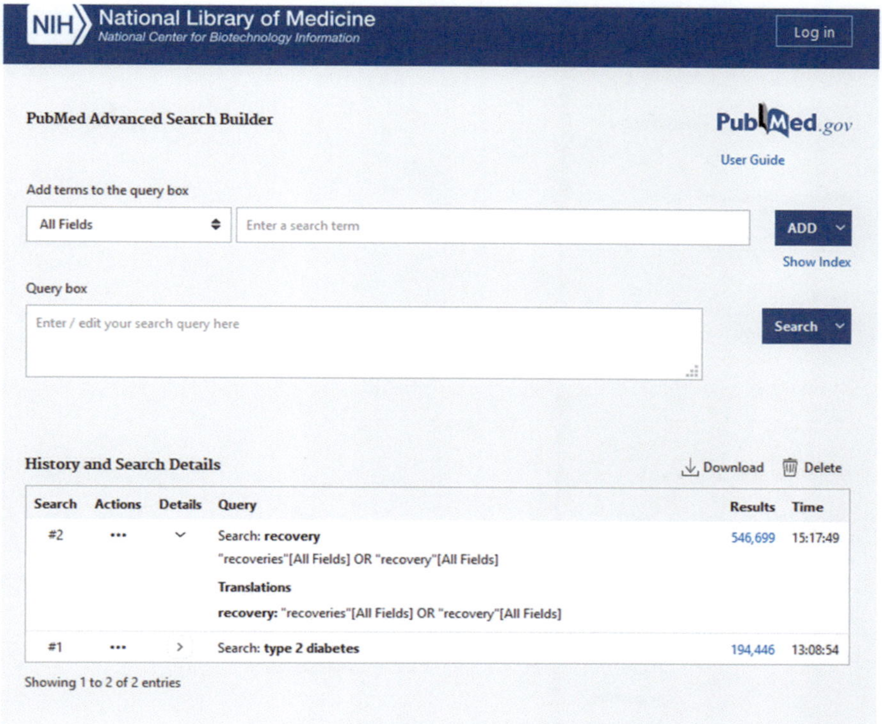

Fig. 3.2 Search Details 2

If you are unable to locate a MeSH term that is relevant, return to PubMed and search using a variety of keywords to capture the various words authors may have used to express the concept. For example, if there is no MeSH term for prehospital care, use *prehospital OR pre-hospital* and consider including related concepts, such as *"Emergency medical services"[MeSH].*

Tip 3: Combine Terms with ANDs and ORs

It is possible to search for all your PICO concepts in one line, such as *obesity AND type 2 diabetes AND bariatric surgery*. However, there may be occasions when you want to search one concept at a time so that you have more clarity and potentially more control over how PubMed is mapping your search terms. In these cases, it is recommended to search one concept at a time using the main PubMed search box on either the PubMed homepage or the PubMed results page and then combine them on the *Advanced* search screen.

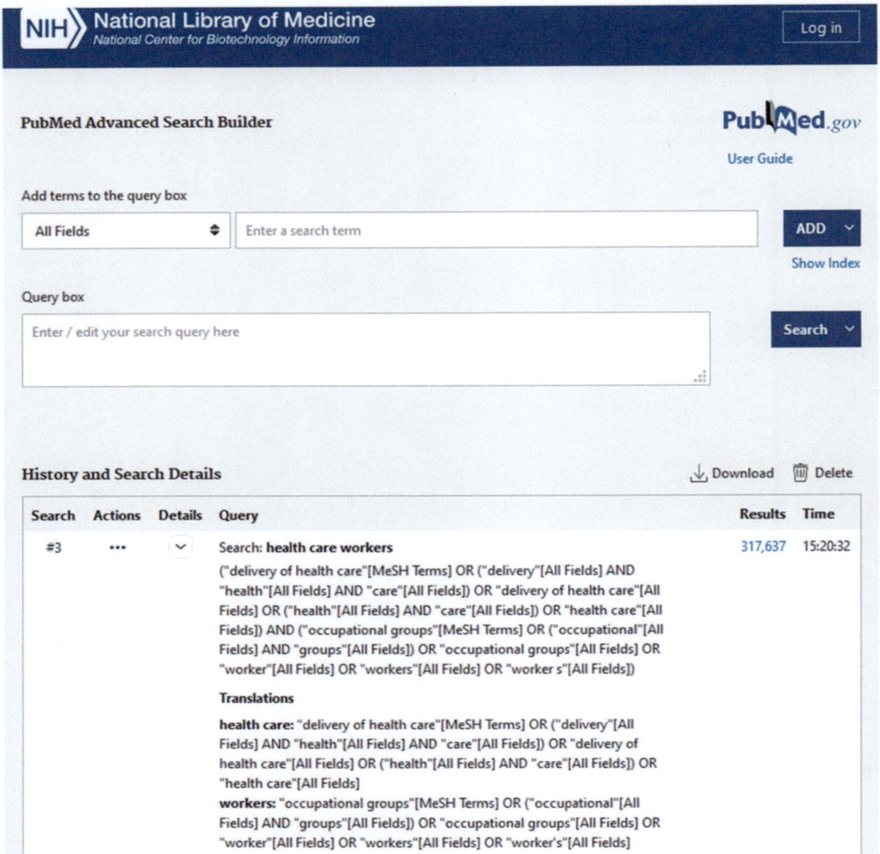

Fig. 3.3 Search Details 3

To combine terms, simply search one concept at a time, confirming that the *Search details* indicate that a relevant MeSH term was included. Each search will be independent, meaning you are not narrowing your search as you go, simply creating separate searches for the different components.

Once you have searches to combine, usually just the Patient problem and Intervention/prognostic factor searches, click on *Advanced*. Your searches should appear in a list as shown in Fig. 3.5.

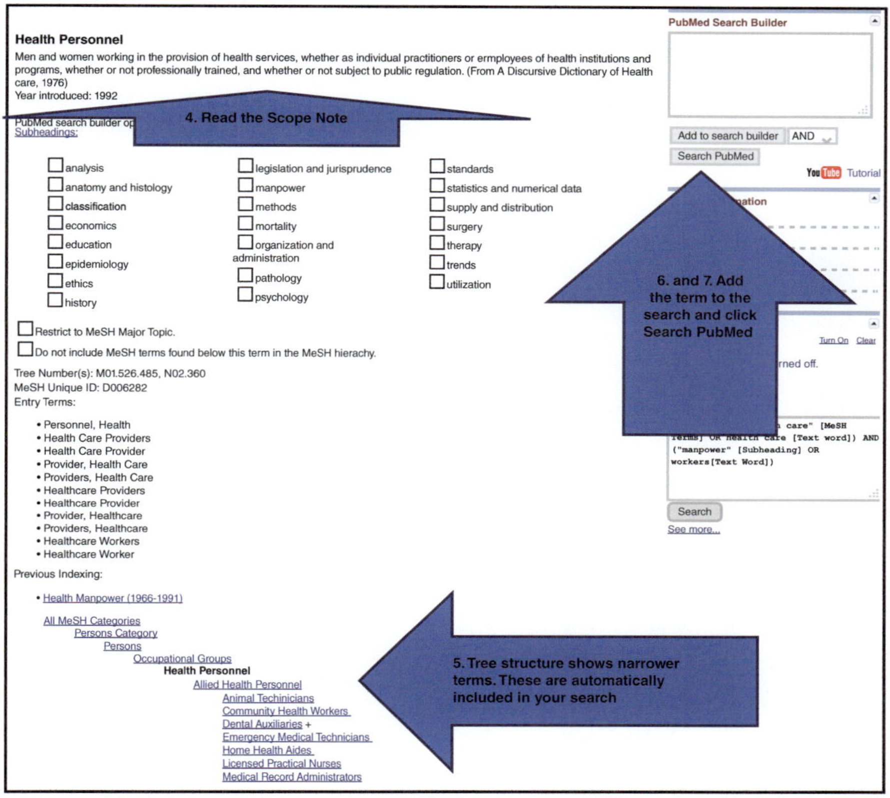

Fig. 3.4 Viewing a MeSH term in the MeSH database

Simply click on the … link under the Actions column for the searches you want to include to move them into the *Query box,* which should result in them looking like the image below in Fig. 3.6.

In this case, we want to *AND* our search concepts together because we want to have results that include all three concepts.

The other primary Boolean operator that can be used as a connecting word is *OR*, depicted in Fig. 3.7. OR is primarily used when you want to find articles that use either term. Remember the recommendation above in tip 3 to search multiple keyword variations when no MeSH term is available? This used OR because it finds articles that may use different words (or even spellings!) for the same concept.

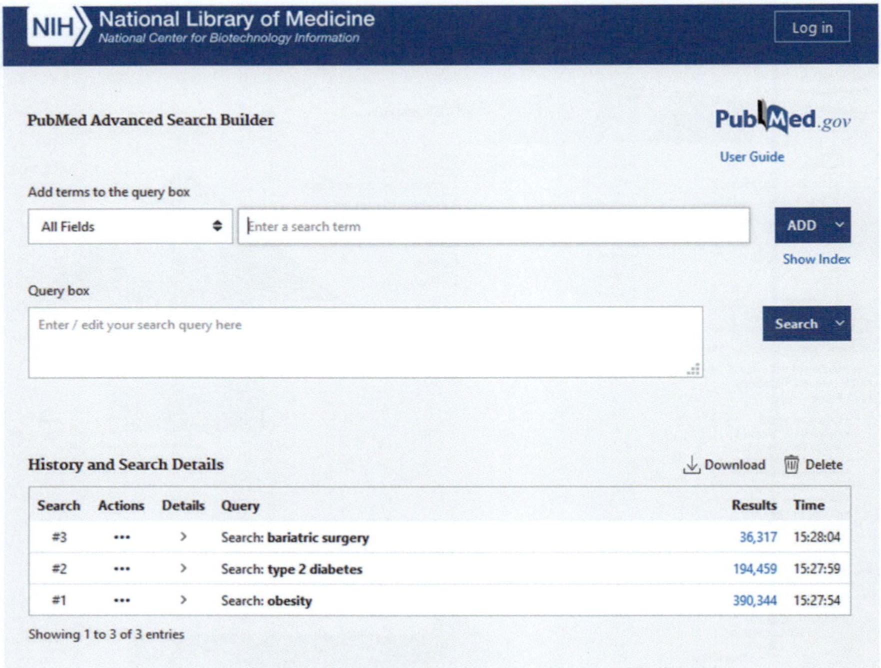

Fig. 3.5 Advanced Search Box

Tip 4: Narrow Your Search to the Best Study Design for the Type of Question You Are Asking

As we discuss in detail in the introduction chapter on clinical questions, certain study designs are better suited for answering the different kinds of clinical questions. Therefore, the last tip for finding the highest quality and most relevant research to address your clinical question, is to narrow your search results to the appropriate type of study, as listed in Table 3.2:

There are two primary ways to narrow your search results: using either the filters on the search results page or the Clinical Queries option.

Search Results Filters: Article types appear as options on the search results filters. By default, only some filters automatically appear, but more can be displayed and selected. These filters are based on publication type categories that are assigned

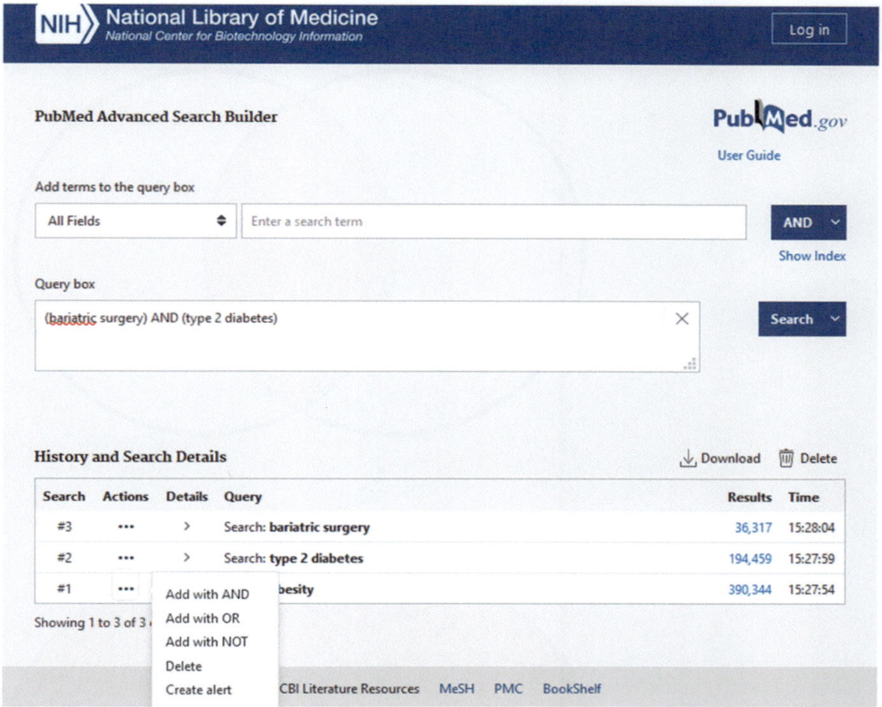

Fig. 3.6 Search Builder

when the article is indexed. Not all of the standard study designs are available as options—notably, cohort study is missing. If you want to narrow to a specific kind of study not included as a publication type filter, consider ANDing it to your search strategy as a MeSH term or keyword.

Clinical Queries: The other option for limiting to certain study types is to use the Clinical Queries filters, found on the homepage of PubMed. These were built based on the primary EBM question types (Therapy, Prognosis, Diagnosis, Etiology, and Clinical Prediction Guides), and use sophisticated search strategies to narrow to the best study designed for each question type. Each filter comes with a Broad or Narrow scope, so that the user can determine if they are willing to go Broad, and perhaps have to sift through some less relevant results, or Narrow, and perhaps miss something that might be relevant.

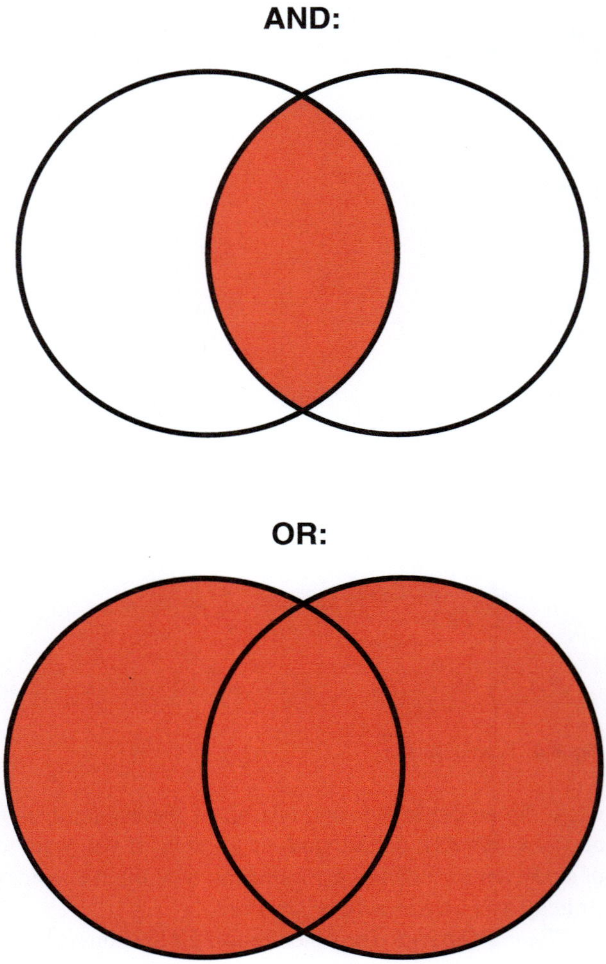

Fig. 3.7 AND vs. OR

Table 3.2 Study designs used to answer different clinical questions

Type of Question	Possible study designs
Diagnostic testing	Cross-sectional, cohort
Therapy or prevention	RCT
Screening	RCT (screening is an intervention, too!)
Causation or harm	RCT > cohort > case control > case series
Prognosis	Cohort > case series
Natural history	Cohort > case series
Prevalence	Cross-sectional
Incidence	Cohort

Clinical Queries can be used for simple searches by simply typing the concepts into the Clinical Queries search box; however this does not allow you to check search details or add MeSH terms from the MeSH database. To use the Clinical Queries after building a more advanced search, a user should:

1. Complete a search building sets as above.
2. Copy the final search strategy using CTRL-C or other browser copy function.
3. Click on the PubMed home screen.
4. Click on Clinical Queries.
5. Paste the final search strategy using CTRL-V or other browser paste function into the Clinical Queries search box.
6. Select the Category based on clinical question type.
7. Select the Scope for Broad or Narrow based on a review of results.

To simplify this process, users can add the Clinical Queries as filters on their own PubMed results screen using the NCBI customization features. These filters appear on the left side of search results and can be highly customized to user preferences. In addition to adding the Clinical Queries, users can add filters for age groups, specific journals, and other options. Additional information on adding filters is available in the My NCBI Help book online at https://www.ncbi.nlm.nih.gov/books/NBK53591/

> Click on the icon next to *My NCBI Filters* at the top of the filters options and sign in.
> You can select from the lists of *Popular, LinkOut, Properties, Links*, or *Search* to find filters.
> Check the filter you would like to add.
> Your filters will appear when you return to your PubMed results.

Tip 5: Selecting an Article

Regardless of resource used to conduct a search, once you have completed a search, you should have a set of articles of varying relevance to your clinical question and patient. How do you choose which is best?

It is rare to find an article (and only one article) that studied a group of patients that exactly matches your own, so be prepared to sift through some results and to select articles based on what is most important to your patient. Consider changing the *Sorted by* display of your results from *Best Match* to *Most Recent* and vice versa to see both relevant and new articles towards the top of your results list. Consider the relevance of the article to your PICO question, the generalizability of the patients in the research study to your own patient, the date the article was published, and what journal published the article. Be aware that some older articles remain the gold standard and most timely research on a topic, so narrowing just to the most recent

5 years may not be appropriate. Similarly, not every article in the "best journals" is going to be the best article. You will need to use your judgment in appraising the content of the article, not just the name of the journal that published it.

Streamlining Your Searches

Working with Results: Google Scholar, Scopus, and Other Primary Resources

There are many tools in Google Scholar, Scopus, and other resources that allow you to work with results. While PubMed offers filters to narrow by age, gender, and type of study (as above), other databases such as Google Scholar and Scopus, have different filtering options. Notably, neither Google Scholar nor Scopus allows you to filter by study type, which make them challenging to use for focused clinical questions. The closest way to filter to the evidence is to type the kind of study as part of the search strategy, such as bariatric surgery and type 2 diabetes and obesity and randomized controlled trial. Be aware that other resources offer different defaults and choices for sorting, often defaulting to either newest or most relevant articles, which sometimes ends up being older review articles. In Scopus, the default is to sort by publication date, but there is the choice to also sort by other options, including times cited. This feature, which is not available in PubMed, allows you to quickly identify articles that have been cited many times. This can be a good strategy for identifying older landmark trials.

Saving Your Work

To streamline your searches in PubMed, sign up for an NCBI account. As referenced in the above section on *Clinical Queries*, NCBI accounts allow you to create your own filters for narrowing results. In addition, NCBI accounts allow you to save searches and get email alerts when new articles are added on your topic (Box 3.3). Finally, NCBI accounts allow you to save individual article citations in *Collections*. This feature can be useful if there are a standard set of guidelines or articles that you use regularly on a certain service.

Box 3.3 Saving a Search Strategy

From the Results screen, click on *Create alert* below the search box.
Sign in to *NCBI*, if you are not already.
Review the search strategy for accuracy.
Enter a new name for the search and click *Save*.
Select *No* or *Yes* to receive email updates.
If *Yes*, fill in the form indicating how often to get updates, the result format, and the number of items to send.
To access, delete, or edit settings of a search, sign into *NCBI* and click on *Manage Saved Searches*.

Saving Selected Citations

After running a search, select the citations that you would like to save from the Results list by placing a checkmark in the box next to the citation.

Using the *Send to* dropdown menu above the results, select *Collections*.

Select whether you would like to create a new collection for the citations or add them to an existing collection.

Click on *Add*.

Enter a name for your new collection or choose an existing collection from the dropdown menu. Click *Save*.

To access, delete, or share collections, sign into *NCBI* and click on *Manage Collections*.

Regardless of the resource you search, you should be able to download citations to save them into a citation manager like EndNote, Zotero, or Mendeley. Most of these citation managers have desktop- and mobile device-based apps that allow to carry your favorite articles around with you, saving you time and increasing your access to research you need frequently. These tools offer several advantages: they can store the PDF, organize files, save comments/highlights on PDFs, format bibliographies and cited references in Word, and even share libraries.

TEACH IT!!

Teaching learners how to perform effective literature searches is best done in an experiential way. Ideally, all learners will have their own computers or tablets that they can use to conduct their own search.

5 min: Start with a demonstration.

- In context of morning report style case conference—Librarian or presenting resident demonstrates a quick search within context of existing morning report. This is a demonstration only. Librarian and/or residents should show different resources based on question, which allows a variety of resources to be covered over a number of weeks/days.
- In context of EBM course—each topical session should have a case. Ask participants to frame case as PICO question. Teacher/librarian demonstrates quick search for that case.

15–30 min.

This approach gets learners more involved

- In context of morning report—Hand out devices or use participants' own devices to have everyone search for an answer to a clinical question in an existing morning report. Agree to same question ahead of time. Work as individuals, pairs, or groups. Complete a card identifying the citation/resource that answers the question and justify why. Presenting resident/librarian shows answers and facilitates discussion about paths there and results.

- In context of EBM course—each topical session should have a case. Ask participants to frame case as PICO question and find a resource that answers question. Report back and share tips/guidance/feedback.

30–60 min

- Demonstration and learner's own case. 15 min demonstration by instructor, followed by example, then learners' own cases.
- Searching bootcamp—no demonstration. Have five clinical cases max per hour, have people search, then demonstrate/offer tips/guidance.
- Lightning round—no demonstration. Have ten ready reference questions max per hour. Pass the hat and have individuals select a case to search or have everyone search for them all. Instructor should offer tips to improve resource selection and utilization.

60–90 min.

This approach involves full learner engagement and is recommended whenever the learner will be expected to report back on the answer to their clinical question. Any course in EBM which is self-contained and lasts longer than one day can involve learners asking and answering their own clinical questions, and reporting back to the group in brief or extended formats.

- Bring Your Own Case: Learners are prompted to bring their own recent clinical questions or are offered time to reflect on recent cases that inspired questions. Learners develop PICO, select a resource, and conduct a search. Instructor circulates through room to offer individual guidance.

Therapy: Assessing the Value of Clinical Interventions

4

Daniella A. Zipkin, Matthew Tuck, Kathleen W. Bartlett, and Zackary D. Berger

Guide for the Teacher

Therapy is often considered the most important and fundamental of the teaching topics in courses for evidence-based medicine. Therapy questions comprise the bulk of learners' needs in clinical settings, and therapy studies make up approximately 75% of the research literature. Teaching therapy can occur in the beginning or middle of a course, either as the first core topic or embedded within a clinical framework moving from diagnosis to therapy to

Supplementary Information The online version contains supplementary material available at [https://doi.org/10.1007/978-3-031-11174-7_4].

D. A. Zipkin (✉)
Department of Medicine, Duke University Health System, Duke University School of Medicine, Durham, NC, USA
e-mail: daniella.zipkin@duke.edu

M. Tuck
Department of Medicine, Veterans Affairs Medical Center, Medical Service, George Washington University, Washington, DC, USA
e-mail: Matthew.Tuck@va.gov

K. W. Bartlett
Department of Pediatrics, Duke Children's Hospital, Duke University, Durham, NC, USA
e-mail: katy.bartlett@duke.edu

Z. D. Berger
Division of General Internal Medicine, Department of Medicine, John Hopkins School of Medicine, Baltimore, MD, USA
e-mail: zberger1@jhmi.edu

D. A. Zipkin (ed.), *Teaching Evidence-Based Medicine*,
https://doi.org/10.1007/978-3-031-11174-7_4

prognosis. We recommend covering the following components when teaching therapy:

1. Framing a therapy question.
2. Selecting the optimal study design. Study selection is covered separately in the chapter on "Searching the Medical Literature."
3. Assessing the risk of bias in randomized controlled trials of interventions.
4. Calculating absolute risk, absolute risk reduction, relative risk, relative risk reduction, and number needed to treat.
5. Applying results of therapy trials to individual patients.
6. Communicating results of therapy trials to patients.

For each of these sub-topics you will find:

- Core content handout—we recommend learners read ahead of class.
- Samples of articles and accompanying worksheets for exercises to do together during teaching.
- Supplementary material in some cases.
- Links to videos with examples of real time teaching.

While framing the question and selecting the design can be taught in a brief introduction (under 15 min), each of the other topics can comprise an hour of time—risk of bias, therapy math, applying results, and communicating results.

Framing the Question

Evidence based medicine takes place in the context of patient care, and requires individualized attention to the patient's unique situation. When you see a patient, often many questions come to mind. For example, "how does treatment x compare to y in patients with a certain disease." We need to be able to frame our clinical questions in a way that facilitates effective searches of the medical literature and decide whether to apply the results of our literature search to the patient when taking into account their values and preferences. We have reviewed the framing of clinical questions previously in the introductory chapter, and now we will apply the idea to questions regarding therapy.

Anatomy of a Question

> *P* = *Population* (Which patients or problem? Be specific!)
> *I* = *Intervention* (or *exposure* or *test* or *prognostic* factor).
> *C* = *Control or comparison*, if appropriate.
> *O* = *Outcomes* (What is the clinical goal?)

We can specify each component of the question based upon the clinical scenario. Let us use an example: You are seeing a 16-year-old patient in clinic for follow-up of an acute asthma exacerbation. The patient received a single dose of dexamethasone in the emergency department yesterday as opposed to the typical 5-day burst of prednisone you are used to prescribing. You are wondering if this patient received enough systemic steroids. Let us form the PICO for this case:

- Not enough info: "what is the best steroid dose for asthma exacerbation in children?"
- Better:
  - P = children with asthma exacerbation.
  - I = single dexamethasone dose.
  - C = five day oral steroid dose.
  - O = resolution of symptoms.

Now for a second case: Your patient is a 32-year-old woman G1P1 who endured moderate hyperemesis gravidarum in her first pregnancy. She took ondansetron in the past with minimal relief. She is planning a second pregnancy and would prefer to avoid taking pills if possible. She is asking you the value of acupuncture as a treatment for hyperemesis. How might you frame that question?

- Not enough info: "what is the best treatment for hyperemesis gravidarum in pregnancy?"
- Better: "how does acupuncture compare to anti-emetics for the treatment of hyperemesis gravidarum?"
  - P = pregnant women with hyperemesis gravidarum.
  - I = acupuncture.
  - C = oral antiemetics.
  - O = relief of hyperemesis.

Let us try one more case. You are rounding in the cardiac intensive care unit and two fellows are discussing ezetimibe. One fellow believes we should add it to the standard regimen of a statin for anyone leaving the CCU after an acute coronary event. The other fellow says "the studies about ezetimibe are bogus." What is a medical resident to do? Frame the question!

- Not enough info: "should this patient with recent MI take ezetimibe?"
- Better: "should this patient with an acute MI take ezetimibe in addition to a statin in order to further reduce cardiovascular events?"
  - P = patients who have recently undergone acute coronary syndrome.
  - I = ezetimibe added to statin therapy.
  - C = statin therapy alone.
  - O = recurrent coronary events, death, revascularization.

Now, you construct the PICO! You are treating a 65-year-old man with hypertension, diabetes type II, and congestive heart failure with aspirin, lisinopril, carvedilol, atorvastatin, and insulin glargine. His A1c at this appointment is 6.2% and you are both thrilled—he had been trying hard to get it lower. It was previously averaging 7.5%. You wonder what the goal A1c to improve cardiovascular outcomes should be in a patient like him.

- Try this one: "In type II diabetic patients with cardiovascular risk factors, does intensive glycemic control to an A1c below 6.5% improve cardiovascular outcomes?"
  - P =
  - I =
  - C =
  - O =

After framing your question, you will search the literature by using the terms most specific to the question. Often, we leave out terms like "placebo" and the "outcome" terms in our search because they are broad and not specific to just our question. We can let the outcomes emerge in what we find. Literature searching is covered in full in a separate chapter.

Assessing the Risk of Bias

"Therapy" refers to ANY intervention—this could be a medication or procedure, behavioral counseling or screening test. When studying interventions, the best design, when available and possible, is often a *randomized controlled trial (RCT)*. An RCT is a true scientific experiment aiming to isolate the intervention in a way that controls for all other variables, so that the only difference between the two groups you are comparing in the study is the intervention.

Our goal is to determine if a study regarding therapy has drawn conclusions that are valid and applicable to our patient. *Bias* refers to any factor which directs the investigator away from the truth [1, 2]. Bias takes a direction away from the truth—it is a systematic error that skews results in one direction, because of methodological issues built in to the study (in other words, not occurring at random). Bias comes in many forms at every stage of a study, from design and recruitment all the way to analyzing results. Each of the criteria we discuss here is an attempt to minimize the impact of bias on the results of a study. Before a study gets started, we must consider the type of patient that is willing to participate in a trial to begin with. Do these patients generally represent yours? Consider *volunteerism bias*, or the tendency of volunteers to be healthier than average. This impacts generalizability, or the ability to apply the results to a realistic group of patients. Additionally, every treatment confers a *patient burden* which actual patients may not be able to tolerate as research volunteers do.

There are always prognostic patient variables that we cannot account for (a.k.a. confounders), and the method which distributes these variables evenly across groups is called *randomization* [3]. When patients are not randomized, intangible variables (often unmeasurable ones—variables you cannot necessarily adjust for later) will differ between the groups and introduce bias into the results. Randomization means that every subject entering a trial has an equal opportunity to end up in either the intervention or the control group. It should be *computerized*, or utilize a random number generator, and *concealed* from all subjects and investigators. Humans are notoriously bad at ensuring true randomness! *Concealing randomization* means that investigators or study personnel do not know the potential group assignments when they are enrolling patients. Imagine an investigator who just had a patient with a bad outcome due to disease X and believes that patients like them should really be getting active treatment. What happens if they arrange to get those patients into the active treatment arm? Significant bias is introduced, and the equilibration of prognostic factors that we achieve with randomization is severely compromised. When randomization is done well, the experimental and control groups should start out very similarly with regard to demographic variables and clinical variables relevant to the aims of the study. As you might guess, randomization which adheres to computer generated numbers and concealment may still fail to produce comparable groups if the number of subjects is very small—because random variability is more pronounced at smaller group sizes. See also the chapter describing Bias and Random Error for more detail.

Certain variations in the process of randomization deserve mention: *stratification* and *block randomization* [3]. *Stratification* refers to selecting a variable ahead of time which investigators expect will have a major impact on the results or represents a clinically important discrepancy that investigators will explore in a sub-group analysis later. The process of stratification involves dividing the group into those with and without that variable, and then randomly assigning the members of each group to the arms of the study. In this way, randomization and evening out of known and unknown variables between the groups is maintained, with the added benefit of specifically balancing those participants with and without the variable among both the intervention and the control groups. At the end of the study, one can look at the data in sub-groups with and without this variable, and any differences in how the intervention played out in each group are less vulnerable to bias, because of the stratification beforehand. For instance, we might imagine a statin trial stratified by the LDL of the entering participants, such that those below and LDL of 125 and those above an LDL of 125 are randomized separately. At the end of the study, if you see a benefit of the statin only in the group above 125 and not the group below

125, it suggests a potential true differential effect of the intervention depending on LDL. Stratification can be done for more than one variable, so long as the size of each resulting group of patients is sufficient. The statistical process of establishing this group size is beyond the scope of this text.

Block randomization refers to a system of numbered blocks built into the randomization scheme wherein participants are placed in one group or the other in one block at a time, with each block containing an equal and random assortment of the group assignments. Block randomization achieves numeric balance between intervention groups and is particularly important when group sizes are small. As an example, consider "permuted blocks of four," which is a frequently utilized block approach. Permuted blocks of four means that, if group assignments are labeled A and B, the blocks may look something like this: AABB, ABAB, ABBA, BABA, BBAA, and so forth. As blocks are shuttled through in random order, and the process is done by computer, participants are randomly assigned to group A or B as they come through. Most importantly, any site recruiting only a small number of participants will also maintain balance between the groups. This technique is very useful for multi-site trials or any situation where one center is likely to have low enrollment numbers, to maintain the balance at each site. If numbers of participants at each site are low, it is not enough to only stratify by site, since simple randomization after stratifying may still yield imbalanced numbers by random error. Adding the block technique ensures equal numbers between groups. If balance is NOT maintained at each site, then the site itself can become a confounding variable.

Let us also think about the *comparison group* for a moment. If, per chance, the comparator group were to receive a therapy known to be inferior to the intervention in some way, this would stack the deck in favor of the intervention, i.e. confer a systematic bias [4]. While it may seem ridiculous to imagine a study would be set up with this sort of favoritism, it does happen in subtle ways. For instance, esomeprazole, an enantiomer of omeprazole, was studied against omeprazole in several trials in a way that favored esomeprazole—subjects in the esomeprazole group received 40 mg tablets, while subjects in the omeprazole group received 20 mg tablets [5]. Since there is no biologic reason to see a difference between enantiomers, this stacked the deck in esomeprazole's favor, and data such as these can be used to extend patents and reap more revenue for drug companies. Therefore, while it is not traditionally listed in critical appraisal worksheets, the *choice of comparator* deserves our attention!

During the course of the study, patients in both groups should have *equal treatment* with respect to all other variables and clinical treatments. If one group has, for example, more study nurse visits to explain the intervention than the other group, then the nurse visits themselves become a *co-intervention*, or something running in parallel to the intervention that might account for differences seen later, including outcomes.

Blinding, or *masking* patients, investigators, outcome adjudicators, and analysts to the group assignment, is a key part of minimizing bias. When participants are aware of the group to which they are assigned, all of their conscious and unconscious assumptions and expectations play into how they do. In some instances, blinding participants is not possible, but investigators should maximize the parts of the study that can be blinded. Some studies take blinding a step further, and have participants guess the group to which they were assigned, to demonstrate if unintentional un-blinding may have occurred during the study (for instance, if there are physiologic effects of the intervention that may have been clues to participants). Lack of blinding has a greater impact on study outcomes when those outcomes are subjective, such as symptom scores or self-reported health status, because subjective outcomes reflect participants' attitudes and state of mind. While lack of blinding is less likely to impact objective outcomes such as clinical events, participants' tendency to present to clinical care for symptoms in the first place may still be impacted.

Complete *follow-up* is another important part of minimizing bias. If a large proportion of participants are lost to follow-up, outcomes may be biased by unevenness between the study groups in the characteristics of people who followed through to the end, compared to those who drop out. This can compromise the balance achieved by randomization. There is no "cutoff" for an acceptable amount of loss to follow-up, but over 20% should be cause for concern. Investigators have several options for managing the data of those lost to follow-up. One common method is to carry the last available data point forward to the end and analyze that way. Naturally, some who would have had different outcomes had they continued on will be missed.

The preferred manner for analyzing the results is using a method called *intention-to-treat* [6]. This means that we analyze subjects according to the group to which they were originally randomized, even if they end up receiving the treatment the opposite group did. Why do we do this? To preserve everything we have worked so hard to maintain up until this point! Remember the goal of randomization is to assure equal chance of receiving the intervention or the comparison, thereby distributing all potential confounders evenly between the two groups. When people choose not to take the intervention to which they were assigned, their reasons for doing this (which we cannot possibly surmise) are confounding variables. Thus, if we analyze subjects according to the treatment they actually receive, this destroys this principle of randomization. Using an intention-to-treat analysis or analyzing patient outcomes as we "intended to treat" them reflects care in the real world, where adherence is never guaranteed. Intention-to-treat analyses do tend to underestimate the effect of the intervention or exposure, because some degree of crossover is likely present in the study. This potentially biases the study towards the null hypothesis, or, stated another way, makes it harder to find a difference if one is really there. However, if a difference is found, it is likely a robust one. There are a number of alternative analyses which do not follow the principle of intention to treat, and they may go by a variety of names, including "per protocol" analysis, "efficacy" analysis, "as treated" analysis. Figures 4.1 and 4.2 show the differences between intention to treat analyses and per protocol analyses.

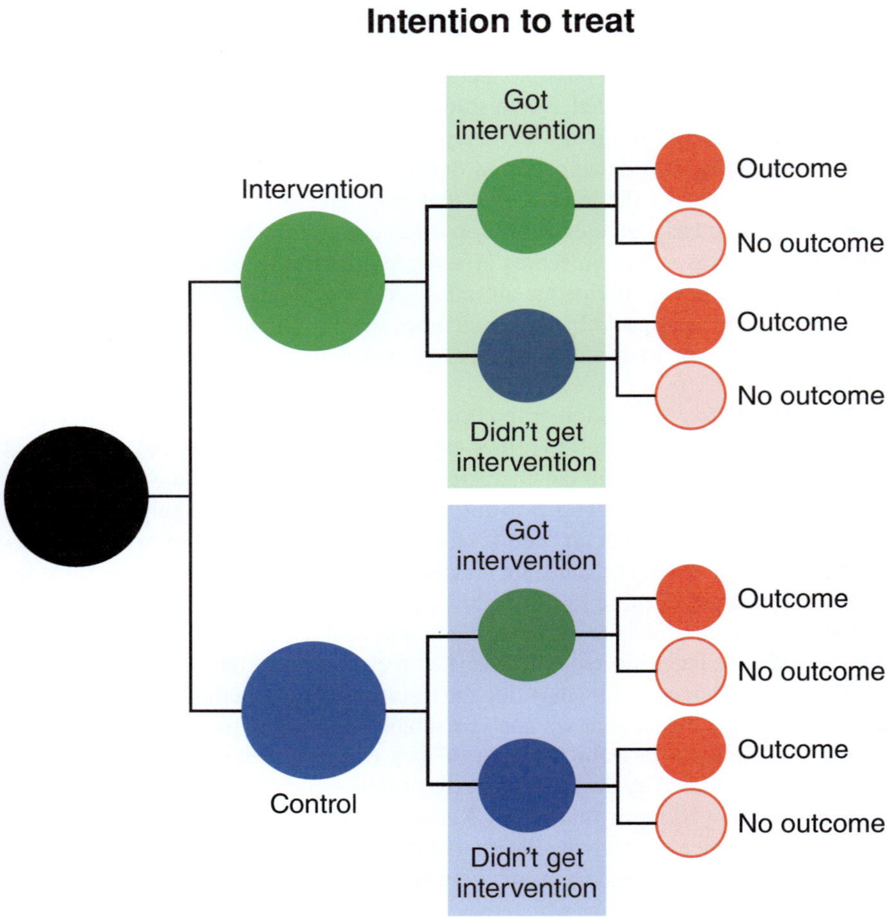

Fig. 4.1 Intention to Treat Analysis

An intention to treat analysis is one in which participants are analyzed in the group to which they were randomized, regardless of whether they stayed with that assigned intervention. In this diagram in Fig. 4.1, all of those in the green shaded box are analyzed in the intervention group, and all of those in the blue shaded box are analyzed in the control group.

In Fig. 4.2, those shaded green are analyzed in the intervention group, and those shaded blue are analyzed in the control group. Notice the analysis will not match participants as they were assigned, but according to the treatment they received—allowing in biases, since the investigators cannot account for the reasons this may have happened.

Sometimes investigators will conduct a *"run-in"* phase to assess compliance in their entire group *before* they randomize. This essentially provides a population

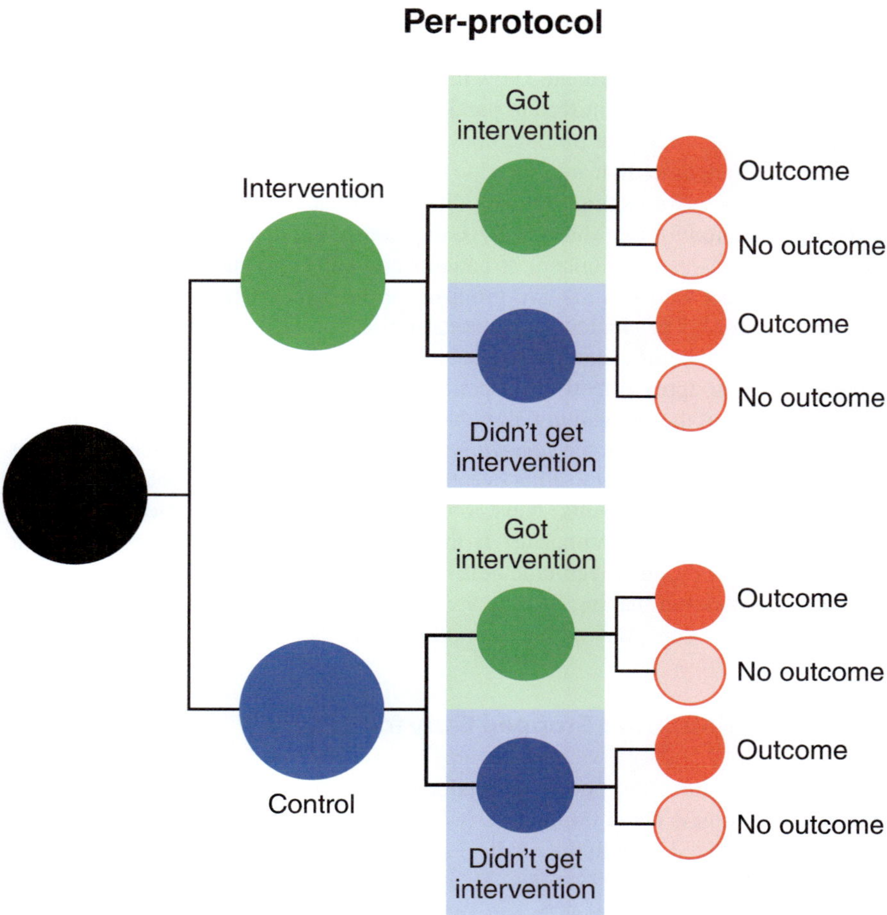

Fig. 4.2 Per Protocol Analysis

with a lower expected non-compliance rate, so that more randomized subjects are actually receiving the prescribed treatment, and the treatment effect can be larger. Because this happens prior to randomization, it does not compromise the intention-to-treat principle. However, we may not be able to generalize these results to our patients, who better reflect the larger population, before the run-in phase removed the less compliant patients.

In assessing the value of a study in informing your patient care, it is also important to note which *outcomes* were measured. *Surrogate endpoints*, such as FEV-1 or lipid profiles, for example, may not tell you what you ultimately want to know about morbidity and mortality. Surrogate outcomes are chosen because they are easier to measure, require shorter follow-up, and correlate with an outcome of interest. In assessing a surrogate outcome, one must be certain that there is a strong, independent and consistent association between the surrogate endpoint and the clinical endpoint of interest. Ideally, we would like to know that there are randomized trials showing that the surrogate outcome has moved in parallel with the target outcome.

Another common format for outcomes is the *composite outcome*. Composites are collections of outcomes that are related to the condition of interest but differ in severity and frequency (for example, major adverse cardiac event, cardiovascular death, and hospitalization for a cardiac event). Using composite outcomes allows investigators to enroll reasonable numbers of patients and still have enough events occur to show a difference between the two groups (see the discussion of power which follows this section). The challenge with interpreting composite outcomes is that each component of the composite may not contribute equally to the results, and they are more difficult to apply directly to a patient. To approach a report with composite outcomes, look at the individual risk reduction of each component of the composite and first see if they move in the *same direction*. Does one outcome worsen while others improve? Is the *frequency* of the events similar across the composite, or does one piece seem to be driving results? Next, look at the *magnitude* of the effect—is it similar across pieces of the composite? If the components are similar with regard to direction, frequency, and magnitude, it is likely safe to use the composite outcome as the basis for decision making. If they are not, then consider looking at the components separately—recognizing that their individual power is limited.

Truncated Trials: Trials Stopped Early for Benefit

One important and often poorly understood situation where random error comes into consideration is *trials stopped early for apparent benefit*. These studies tend to be highly publicized in both the medical and lay media and more rapidly applied to clinical practice than other studies. However, because they are reporting conclusions based on fewer observed events than originally planned, they run the risk of vastly *overestimating treatment effects*. They might just be "too good to be true."

Here is a list of questions to ask yourself when considering the results of a truncated trial:

- *Was there a pre-specified stopping rule* and was the boundary of statistical significance stringent (i.e., $p < 0.001$)? Checking the data frequently to look for the event rate to cross a certain boundary leads to a higher chance of spurious findings.
- *Were there a large number of outcome events?* The fewer the events in the trial, the greater the chance of an inflated estimate of treatment effect. Fewer than 200 events leaves the greatest chance of spurious findings. Greater than 500 events, on the other hand, is the more reliable in leading to a true estimate of effect [7].
- Were results of *other studies on the same topic* similar in their conclusions?

A visual depiction of trials stopped early is provided in Fig. 4.3.

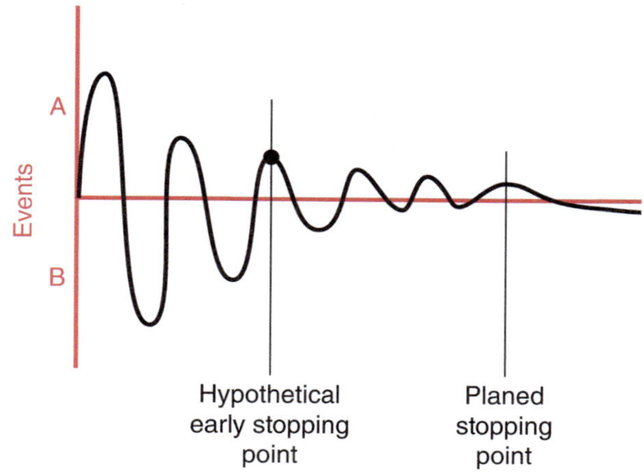

Fig. 4.3 Trials Stopped Early for Benefit

Events do not accrue evenly in both groups across the span of a trial. The wavy line represents uneven event accrual as time progresses, in intervention group A and control group B. When the trial is stopped early, it runs the risk of seeing an effect size that is inflated because of the spurious accumulation of events in each group. Event rates based on a smaller number of events than planned will risk being erroneous, due to chance (Box 4.1).

Box 4.1 Minimizing Bias in Studies of Therapy

1. Was randomization carried out, via objective, computerized process? Was the allocation of subjects to randomly determined groups concealed? Did the intervention and control groups subsequently have similar proportions of prognostic variables?
2. Were subjects, investigators, statisticians, and outcome adjudicators blinded to treatment group?
3. Were the study groups treated equally, aside from the intervention of interest?
4. Was follow-up as complete as can be reasonably expected?
5. Was an intention-to-treat analysis performed?
6. If the trial was stopped early, did investigators adhere to a pre-specified stopping threshold while maintaining statistical rigor?

Error in Clinical Trials

Before we assess treatment effects, we should make sure we believe the results of the trial. Think of the trial as a diagnostic test, trying to "diagnose the truth"—how close the trial gets to telling us the true state of affairs. A number of errors can occur along the way, as illustrated in Table 4.1.

Table 4.1 Error in clinical trials

	TRUTH—Drug A really is better than Drug B	TRUTH—Drug A really is not better than Drug B
Trial says—Drug A is better than Drug B	True positive	False positive (α, type I error)
Trial says—Drug A is not better than Drug B	False negative (β, type II error)	True negative

$$\text{Type I error} = \text{risk of false positive} = \alpha = \text{the } p-\text{value.}$$

The *p*-value is the probability of a false positive conclusion. Therefore, the smaller the *p*-value, the more confident we are in a true positive.

$$\text{Type II error} = \text{risk of false negative}$$
$$= \beta = \text{a value determined at the beginning of the study.}$$

$$\text{Power} = (1-\beta) = \text{probability of true negative.}$$

If a study finds no difference, we must ask, did it have enough power to find a difference if one was really present? This is analogous to the sensitivity of a diagnostic test. Many studies historically set the β at 0.20—a 20% chance of concluding that there is no benefit when there actually is, or a power of 80%. This convention appears to be changing with many modern studies moving towards a β of 0.10, or 90% power.

Before initiating a study, the investigators must calculate the goal *sample size* using: (1) *the known frequency of events at baseline in their population over a specified time frame*, (2) *the anticipated effect size of the treatment being tested, and* (3) *their chosen* α *and* β. They should state in the article what the goal *sample size* was, and how many *outcome events* are needed from that sample, to maintain their level of power. If they did not calculate this ahead of time, or did not achieve their target sample, power comes into question. *If they achieved the target sample size, but that sample did not reach the expected number of outcome events, they still lack the power they intended.* Ultimately, sample size is important because of the number of outcome events needed, so *outcome events* is the most important factor to look for at the end of the study in determining if power is maintained. Naturally, negative studies which were *stopped early for no difference* are particularly vulnerable to this issue with lack of power, because they will likely have fewer outcome events.

In addition to stopping early, other issues affecting power include *crossover* (or *"contamination")* between experimental groups, and incomplete *follow-up*. Crossover of subjects from one group to another, or contamination, occurs when the experimental or control group receive the intervention intended for the other arm of the study. Imagine, for instance, that the subjects independently seek out the intervention to which they were not randomized. This will make the two groups more similar and make it harder to find a difference in outcomes with the intervention if one were really there. Similarly, increases in loss to follow-up limits the potential outcomes which can be measured, and therefore reduces the overall event rates of the trial—with fewer events, it is harder to find a difference if one is really there.

Interpreting One Small Study in the Universe of Data

When a study has a small number of events to look at, certain issues arise. Small numbers of events can occur for several reasons: the study may have been small to begin with; the investigators were unable to recruit the goal sample size; even with the goal sample size, the number of outcome events was unexpectedly low; or the trial was stopped early (whether with, or without, a pre-specified statistical stopping threshold). We sort the issues involved according to whether the study in question was *POSITIVE* or *NEGATIVE*.

Small positive studies: When a study finds a difference (a *positive* study) between two interventions, but it is based on a small number of events, the biggest concern is for the possibility of *random error* or a *type I error*. When event rates are small, even statistically significant findings can occur by random error. Typically, *trials stopped early (truncated trials)* have fewer events at the time of stopping than initially planned, and should hold the data to a more rigorous statistical threshold than a later comparison. Despite greater statistical rigor, results which meet statistical thresholds can still occur by chance [8]. Trials stopped early run the risk of spurious findings due to random error, unless total event rates reach the 500 range for the trial as a whole [7]. For more discussion of trials stopped early, see the Study Design chapter.

Small negative studies: When a study finds no difference between two interventions (a *negative* study) based on a small number of events, the biggest concern is for the possibility of *lack of power*, or a *type II error*, as discussed above [9]. There are a few things we can check when a small study is negative, to assess if it might have missed an actual difference in effect:

- Look at the confidence interval, which represents the "neighborhood of truth" around the point estimate. In a negative study, the confidence interval crosses the line of no difference. However, if the confidence interval is broad and includes a lot of positive territory, it may be a clue that the study "missed the boat"—that power was not adequate in this study.
- Check the power calculation in the statistics section for the number of events the authors needed to accrue to maintain power—not just the sample size! Then check the main results table to see if that *number of events* was reached.
- Consider whether or not *historical benefits* were maintained in the study. Factors such as the context of care and advances in care will impact whether historical assumptions can be expected to hold today. As care advances overall, the benefit that older therapies saw in the past may be less now. For instance, consider breast cancer. Treatment for breast cancer has advanced tremendously over the past two decades. Any new intervention will have to compete with control groups receiving better overall cancer care than in the past. This type of narrowing of the margin for therapeutic benefit can also compromise power, making it harder to find a difference between groups.

Teach It!!

The following sections contain suggested exercises to help facilitate your teaching of concepts important to therapy questions and randomized controlled trials. We have grouped them according to the approximate amount of time it takes to do the exercise, to help you with planning classroom time. Depending on the demonstration, the preparatory time will vary.

TEACH IT!!

Assessing Bias in Studies of Therapy: Randomization

Additional depictions of the concepts of randomization, block randomization and stratified randomization are available in Video 4.1 *which accompanies this chapter.*

5–10 min:

Begin by asking learners why clinical trials should be randomized. Answers might include to "balance the experimental and control groups," "to reduce bias or confounding" or "to assure groups are similar." The learner may need coaching to arrive at what these statements really mean. Ultimately, explain that the purpose is to balance prognostic factors, both known and unknown, that may affect outcomes.

Ask the group how true randomization can be achieved; correct replies would include "computerized" or "random number generator" or similar.

Ask the group if it would work if you put 50 pieces of paper with "Group A" written on them, and 50 pieces of paper with "group B" written on them, and asked people to sequentially pull out a slip of paper, up to 100 people. If everyone holds onto their own slip of paper and does not return it to the bag, it becomes obvious that the groups will be imbalanced. *This is because each new participant does not have an equal chance of being in either group.*

15–30 min:

Add tools and visual aids to demonstrate the principles of randomization. For example: Candy demonstration—prepare with a multicolored candy ahead of time. Tell the group to imagine that each color is a potential confounding variable, such as gender or co-morbidities. They can flip a coin to determine which group each candy enters (heads for one group, tails for another). Have one half of the group work with a small population, say 20 candies. Have the other half of the group work with a larger population, say 100. Observe how the confounding variables are more balanced after randomization with larger populations.

30–60 min:

Tackle additional concepts related to randomization, such as stratified and block randomization.

Utilize an article that involves stratified randomization. Ask the group why the investigators would stratify based on those factors. Explain that those factors are confounders that are so important that the investigators wanted to ensure that they would be evenly distributed between the study groups. Also, the investigators can look at those subgroups later, and exploring the differences between them is more rigorous than if it were done in a post hoc analysis because they were randomized within those subgroups, so additional confounders should be balanced. Diagram on a white board: total population at the top; two branches coming down from the top forming two groups—one WITH the stratified variable, and one WITHOUT; from there, each node has two branches coming down from it, representing the study groups A and B.

60–90 min:

- Make it experiential: If you have a large group and a minimum of 60 min for this portion, consider creating a real-time randomization experience. Prepare ahead of time by randomly assigning learners to two or more groups with color-coded cards or candies or another small item concealed in opaque envelopes.
- As participants reach the classroom, tell them that they were randomized by computer to one of two groups, and hand them the card or candy. Once everyone is in place in the room, use an overhead projector to see how the randomization scheme worked out. For example, how many girls are in each group, how many people from out of state are in each group, etc. If you are working with a small group, this is a powerful demonstration of how randomization does not always result in equal groups with respect to a variable of interest.
- To demonstrate block or stratified randomization, it is useful to create more than one color designation. Again, this requires preparation; you must first generate a stratified randomization sequence for a list of learners according to things like their age and sex. Then assign color-coded cards with the two different colors to represent the study groups. On the cards, place different stickers to represent a stratified variable of interest on them. Again, use an overhead projector to show how groups appear more equal with respect to the variables of interest. Tell the group that all the participants with a certain color sticker have a comorbidity of interest, say for instance, diabetes. Have all the participants with diabetes stand up. Then, raise hands if they are assigned to group A by the color of their card, or group B. Demonstrate on the overhead projector that stratification kept balance in the groups with respect to the variable of diabetes.

TEACH IT!!

Assessing Bias in Studies of Therapy: Allocation Concealment

5–10 min.

Discuss allocation concealment as a PART of randomization. Once participants are randomized, the process of allocating participants to their groups should be, but is not always, free of bias. The following scenarios will help learners appreciate how bias may enter allocation concealment.

Ask the learner if they can imagine a way in which the allocation of participants to groups could be biased. Ask for their thoughts on why concealing this process is important. Point out that this is different from the blinding of the study itself.

Discuss an example: Imagine that the randomized order in which participants will be enrolled in group A or group B has been prepared by a computer, but the assignments are filed in a long box in paper envelopes. If the envelopes are a little bit translucent, and the investigator has a bias, the investigator could potentially manipulate the make-up of each group. Say the intervention is a diet, and the investigator has a bias that morbidly obese patients won't succeed on this new diet, and shuttles more of them to the comparator group. He does so by holding the envelope to a light each time a patient is enrolled into the study and skipping to the next envelope if the first one places the patient in the intervention (diet) group. This will skew the results seen at the end of the study and severity of obesity will become a confounder—something that differs between the groups.

Another example: Imagine that you are working in the emergency department, and your friend is running a clinical trial of an investigative new antiviral drug for influenza A that has been rumored to reduce mortality from influenza in high risk patients. You diagnose a patient with influenza A, and the patient has comorbidities that make them high risk—diabetes and heart failure. You call the study center to enroll the patient and they tell you "Great! The next assignment for a new participant will be to placebo." Are you likely to still enroll the patient, knowing they will be getting placebo? Maybe not! If we knew ahead of time that someone was going to be in placebo, we might selectively avoid enrolling the patients we are most worried about, resulting in a study population that does not match the patients to whom we'd like to apply the results.

TEACH IT!!

Assessing Bias in Studies of Therapy: Choice of Comparator

This topic is often overlooked in EBM curricula but is critically important. The way a study in constructed impacts what it can find.

10–15 min:

Diagram a basic randomized controlled trial line drawing on the board as in Fig. 4.4. Give an example of a study for illustrative purposes: Imagine you are building a randomized trial to explore whether or not the reported harms of diet soda are true—does diet soda cause diabetes? One randomized group has to get a diet soda product. Ask the learners, "What does the comparator group get"? Learners may suggest water, or regular soda, or nothing. Then, ask them to look at it from different vantage points. What would they pick if they represented a holistic foods organization? Perhaps water as the comparator, to make diet soda look worse. What would they pick if they were a corporation that only manufactured diet soda? Perhaps regular soda, since it's got to be worse! As the learners wrestle with this simplistic example, they will realize there is a tendency to stack the deck in the direction you hope for the results to go, based on the perspective you have. This is not necessarily a conscious process, and it's not necessary to assign blame—only to realize where human weaknesses may play out in the data we see!

Pair this exercise with examples from the literature, where the comparator was not optimal. When this occurs, consider the funding source of the study, and what they had to gain or lose based on how the study was structured.

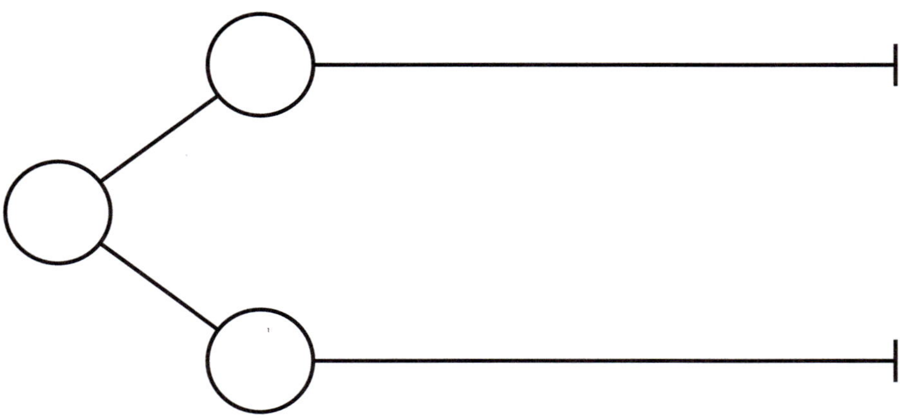

Fig. 4.4 Randomized Controlled Trial

TEACH IT!!

Assessing Bias in Studies of Therapy: Blinding/Masking

5–10 min:

"Double blind" is a commonly used term in describing studies meant to indicate blinding of the subjects and investigator, but it is actually not quite sufficient as we can never be sure who was blinded unless the authors of the study explicitly state who was blinded. Ask the learners who should be blinded in the course of the study. A full answer should include the investigators, the study personnel, the participants, the outcome adjudicators and the data analysts. The more who are blinded, the less the risk for bias.

In the context of a study you are reviewing, ask the learners what might happen if subjects were aware of their group assignment. Consider that human behavior changes when we have more information. Participants' pre-existing notions of what they expect to happen with a certain treatment may play out, or they may believe it has played out and report that it has. The placebo comparator is there to fight against this natural human tendency!

Keep in mind that blinding is even more critical when the outcome is something subjective, or self-reported, since bias can play into what people report. It has less impact on the results when the outcome is objectively measured and can't be influenced by the patient. (However, keep in mind that even something objective like "myocardial infarction" may be influenced by participants' tendency to seek medical attention, which in turn is influenced by the group to which they believe they are randomized).

It is not always possible to blind participants and investigators. Anytime a treatment causes effects which can be differentiated from the comparator, blinding can't occur. Any time a bias is possible, encourage learners to ask themselves, "in what direction would this tend to push the results?"

For instance, one of the authors of this book has a child with peanut allergy. The child was enrolled in a placebo controlled randomized trial of peanut powder for desensitization of the allergy, and the placebo was an oat powder. The peanut powder did have a faint aroma of peanut, and the child's family was pretty sure they were in the peanut group. When they took their first airplane trip after starting the study, and accidentally left six days' worth of peanut doses behind in their refrigerator, they quickly arranged for a friend to send it to them overnight, at a considerable cost. Would that have happened if they thought they were in placebo? I think not!

Assessing Bias in Studies of Therapy: Equal Treatment

5 min:

This point is best made in the context of a study you are using in your teaching. Ask the learners what might happen if one arm of a study were treated differently—for instance, in a trial of the Mediterranean Diet vs. low-fat diet, the intervention

(Mediterranean Diet) group met with a dietician regularly, while the comparator (low-fat diet) group just got handouts about a low-fat diet. The goal is for learners to conclude that the meetings with the dietitican may constitute a "co-intervention", something aside from the intervention that is having an effect on participants.

Therapy studies: Critical Appraisal

30–60 min:

When you have the opportunity to review a full trial in detail, we recommend using Worksheet 4.0, in the Appendix, as a guide.

Therapy Math

Understanding the Magnitude of the Results

Basic Terms

Keep these definitions in mind as you scan a trial's results section:

$$\text{Odds} = (\text{Number of people with event}) / (\text{Number of people without event}).$$
$$\text{Rate} = (\text{Number of people with event}) / (\text{persons per unit of time}).$$
$$\text{Risk} = (\text{Number of people with event}) / (\text{total number of people}).$$

Generally, if these three measures are calculated for the same data set, then risk will be smaller than odds, because the denominator is larger. See below for more information regarding odds ratios (a ratio of two odds).

Measures of Association [10, 11]

Absolute Risk (AR)—Also known as *event rate*, the proportion of patients in each group suffering an adverse outcome.

Example Let us say old Drug X and new Drug Y are being compared in an RCT over a 5-year period. Drug Y claims to fail less often than Drug X. There are 100 patients in each group. If Drug X leads to 5 bad outcomes and Drug Y leads to 2 bad outcomes, then the absolute risk with Drug X is 5 out of 100, or 5% (i.e., the baseline risk), and the absolute risk with Drug Y is 2 out of 100, or 2% (i.e., the experimental risk).

Once we have two absolute risks for two groups in a study, there are only two mathematical operations we use in EBM to demonstrate their relationship to each other—subtract or divide!

Absolute risk reduction (ARR) "SUBTRACT"—This is the most clinically meaningful number, and represents the absolute difference between the proportion who have the event among controls, and the proportion who have the event among treated patients (the difference between baseline risk and experimental risk). It is the *risk difference*, simply subtraction.

Example The absolute risk reduction of using Drug Y instead of Drug X is 5%–2%, or 3%. You can decide if this is clinically meaningful, depending on the situation. For example, a 3% absolute risk reduction may be viewed as beneficial if the bad outcome Drug Y reduces is mortality in patients with a cancer. It would likely be viewed as less clinically meaningful if Drug Y achieves remission in patients with cancer, but has no change in mortality compared to Drug X.

Relative risk (RR) "DIVIDE"—Also known as the risk ratio. This is the ratio of the risk of events among patients receiving the intervention relative to controls. Risk ratios can be calculated in cohort studies and clinical trials. They CANNOT be calculated in case-control studies for reasons we detail in the Odd Ratio section of "Therapy Math."

Example The relative risk (risk ratio) of using Drug Y is 0.02/0.05, or 0.4.

Relative risk reduction (RRR) (also known as proportional risk reduction)—This is the most commonly reported measure of treatment effect and is expressed as a percent. It is an estimate of the *proportion of baseline risk (the risk in the control group) that is reduced by the therapy*. It is calculated by dividing the absolute risk reduction by the baseline risk in the control group. Because it represents a proportion of baseline risk, it is the primary metric which is "portable"—it can be taken from the summary estimate of a study and applied to your patient's baseline risk in order to see the impact of the intervention on your patient. (Please see the section on Applying Results to Patients). While this is important in our later discussion of applying results to individual patients, relative risk reductions are, on their own, at best inflated, and at worst, deceptive.

RRR can be calculated two ways: (1) 1-RR and (2) ARR/baseline risk. See the following example:

Example The relative risk reduction is ARR/baseline risk, or (5% − 2%)/5%, or 3%/5%, which comes out to 60%. Notice that RRR can also be calculated with 1-RR, or 1-0.4, which is also 60%. The proportion of baseline risk that is reduced by using Drug Y is 60%. This is a much more impressive number than the 3% absolute risk reduction, so you can imagine why relative risk reduction is used more often by researchers reporting the results of their study, as well as companies marketing their drugs. Be cognizant, however, that it may convey less meaning clinically.

What if risk was increased by the intervention? Absolute Risk Increase, or ARI, and Relative Risk Increase, or RRI, are calculated in exactly the same fashion as ARR and RRR. The only difference is that the event rate in question represents harm, instead of benefit.

ARR vs. RRR

These two metrics are both frequently presented in the literature and merit some further discussion of benefits and risks of each. Multiple studies have found that ARR improved patients' understanding of their risk reduction better than RRR [12]. RRR tends to be more persuasive, leading to behavior change, which may be related to an inflated perception of impact of an intervention, since RRR cannot be interpreted accurately without knowing the baseline risk. RRR is particularly risky, therefore, when no baseline risk is provided. Use the Fig. 4.5 to help learners grasp the differences between them.

This simple set of bar graphs demonstrates three hypothetical event rate differences. The ARR and RRR for each is shown, and this can be used as the answer key for the exercise mentioned below in the "teach it" section for ARR and RRR. Learners will see that the same RRR will have very different meanings across different baseline risk, and cannot be interpreted without baseline risk.

Number needed to treat (NNT)—This is the inverse of the ARR. It can be stated as, "the number of patients with the target condition that would need to be treated for the specified period of time to achieve one fewer bad outcome." (We use NNT because it is common language with which to describe the results of any trial. However, we will see later in a discussion of communicating results to patients that it may not be the best choice in that setting.) The higher the NNT, the less clinically meaningful a result becomes, and the greater the chance that side effects will overshadow benefits. In studies of harm, we can calculate the *number needed to harm* (NNH) in the same manner.

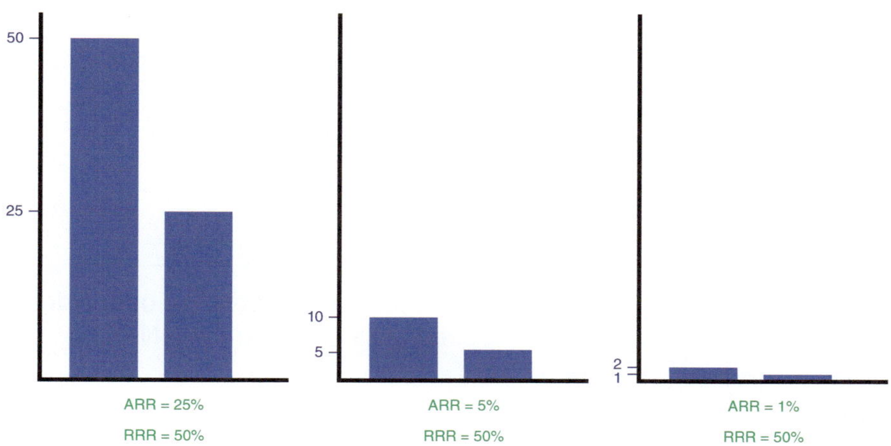

Fig. 4.5 Comparison of ARR and RRR

Example In our original scenario, the ARR was 3%. Therefore, the NNT is 1/0.03 (in decimals), or 100/3 (in percentages), or 33.3. Because we cannot treat a fraction of a person, we round up to 34! This means that we need to treat 34 people with Drug Y instead of Drug X over 5 years to prevent the bad outcome in one person. Reduction of morbidity, cost, and side effects should be considered when deciding how "good" a number needed to treat really is.

Why Does NNT = 1/ARR?

In the examples above, the ARR was 5% − 2%, or 3%. Stated in a sentence, for every 100 patients treated with Drug Y, there are three fewer bad outcomes. So how many patients do we need to treat to prevent one bad outcome? This is the NNT. Dividing both numbers by 3 provides the answer, 33. Note that 100/3 is the same as 1/0.03, or 1/ARR. Figure 4.6 provides a visual depiction of calculating the NNT.

Table 4.2 depicts a 2 × 2 table which can assist in making the calculations above, followed by a box summarizing all of the calculations.

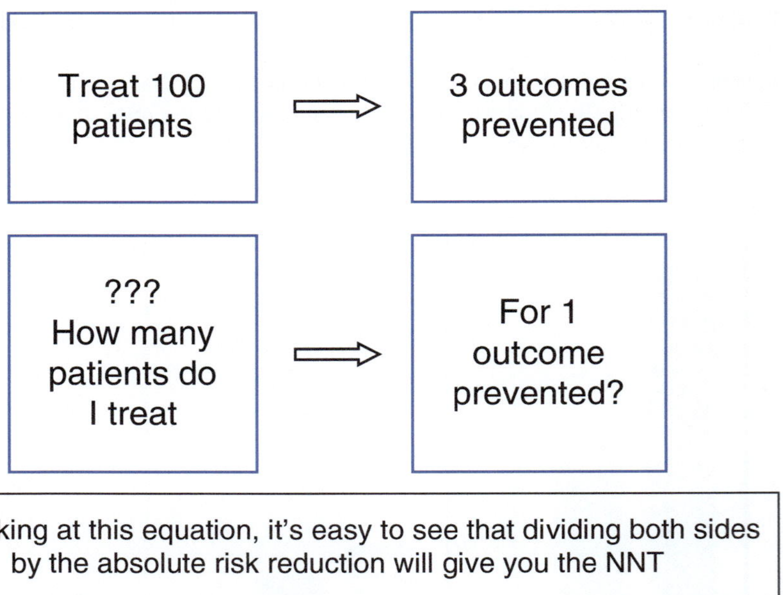

Fig. 4.6 NNT = 1/ARR

Table 4.2 Summary of the math so far

	Outcome—Yes	Outcome—No
Exposure	a	b
No exposure	c	d

RR = "Divide" [a/(a + b)]/[c/(c + d)].
ARR = "Subtract" [c/c + d] − [a/a + b].
RRR = [c/(c + d) − a/(a + b)]/[c/(c + d)] = ARR/baseline risk = 1 − RR.
NNT = 1/ARR (in decimals) or 100/ARR (in percentile).

Odds Ratio (OR) [13]—In contrast to risk, odds is the number of participants having an event divided by the number not having the event. Odds ratios, or a ratio of two odds, represent the odds of having an event in the exposed group divided by the odds of having the event in the control group. Odds ratios are typically seen in case-control studies, where the odds ratio could be the odds of exposure in people with a target disorder versus the odds of exposure in those without a target disorder. (Please see the Introduction chapter, section on study design for a full discussion of these designs.) Odds ratios are calculated in case-control studies because of the nature of the study design. In case control studies there is no concept of "total population" as a denominator as we see in risk ratios, since the investigator is assembling the population from available subjects. Because the investigator is selecting the cases of individuals with a disease or outcome of interest and selecting the controls without a disease or outcome of interest, risk cannot be calculated.

You may also see odds ratios reported in cohort studies and clinical trials. We spend more time reviewing odds ratios in the Harm and Causation section. Because of the way odds are calculated, odds ratios have a smaller denominator and are therefore always larger than risk ratios using the same data. (Please see the chapter on Harm and Causation for more detail on this topic). If you see odds ratios used in clinical trials, ask yourself, "why?"—is there any benefit other than to slightly inflate the number over the risk ratio? Beware of the use of odds ratios which may only serve to make results look more impressive!

	Outcome—Yes	Outcome—No
Exposure	a	b
No exposure	c	d

OR for cohort studies and clinical trials (odds of outcome given certain exposure)
= [a/b]/[c/d] or ad/cb
OR for case-control studies (odds of exposure given certain outcome)
= [a/c]/[b/d] or ad/cb
[Notice that mathematically, these OR calculations start in different places, but come out to be the same!]

Hazard Ratio (HR) [14]—The calculation of a hazard ratio is beyond the scope of this text. However, you should be aware of the general principles upon which they are calculated and be able to interpret them. Generally, studies look at event rates at one point in time, the end of the study. When they look at outcomes over time, however, the data may be described with a *survival curve*. Survival curves represent the status of patients over time. As data accumulate, and certain patients experience the outcome of interest (it may be death, but it may be a new diagnosis—don't be fooled by the "survival" terminology!), the curve represents those remaining in the study, disease free. Naturally, at different points in time, the rate at which subjects remain disease free will change, because the total denominator will change. Statistically, the *hazard ratio* represents the weighted ratio of these rates over the entire course of the study, adjusting for changes over time. The hazard ratio integrates values in small increments over the course of the study and can be thought of as the risk ratio "at any given point in time." A risk reduction can be calculated from the survival curve usually at the end of the study, but the risks at any point in time may look quite different in getting to that point. Therefore, the hazard ratio adds additional information. Imagine curves that balloon out in separate directions but converge towards the end of a study, as in Fig. 4.7. If you do not incorporate the data throughout the study, you

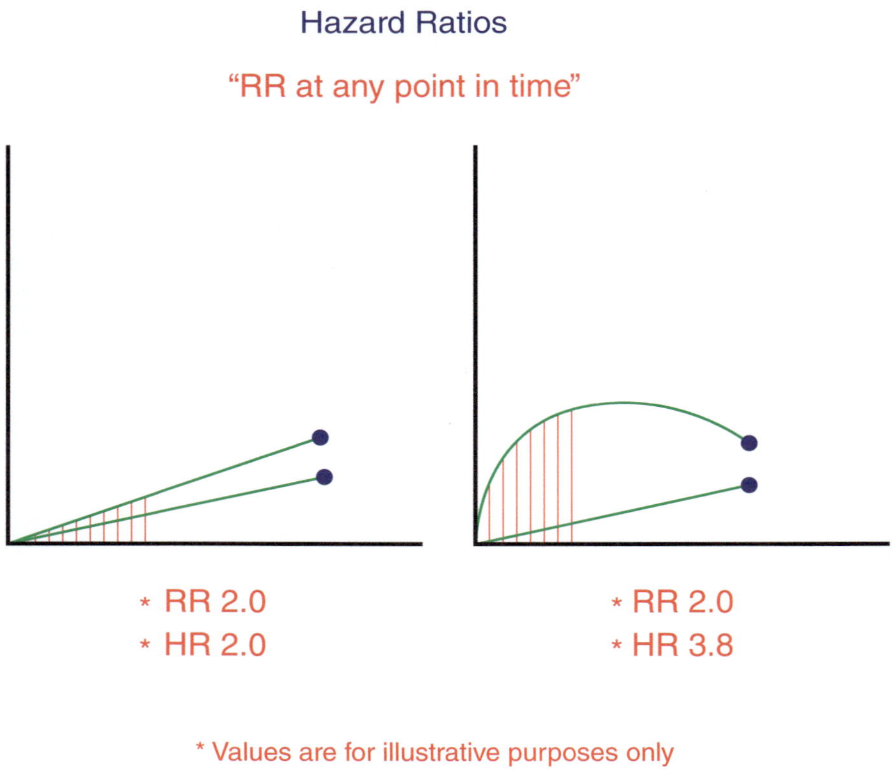

Fig. 4.7 Hazard ratios

may underestimate the true differences between the arms. Hazard ratios are particularly fitting for high risk conditions such as cancer. Imagine a 2-year study of a new drug for end stage cancer. All of the patients have a poor prognosis at the time of enrollment, and at the end of the trail, all subjects are deceased. However, if most patients in the control group die in the first 6 months, whereas the treatment group mostly survives for the first 18 months of the study, the treatment may be beneficial even though the curves converge at the end. Video 4.2 which accompanies this chapter also includes a discussion of visual aids for hazard ratios

We use a schematic illustration of simplified survival curves where one is linear and one has obvious early differences, but they end up at the same event rate by the end of the study time period. The hazard ratio may be similar to the risk ratio in linear data, illustrated by the curve on the left, but differ greatly from the risk ratio in non-linear data, illustrated by the curve on the right. Hazard ratios integrate risk ratios across infinitesimally small intervals to provide a more accurate depiction of the risk ratio across the entire scope of the study period. This diagram can be used in any Harm or Therapy teaching, as a quick visual for learners to grasp why a study is presenting results as a Hazard Ratio.

How Precise Is the Treatment Effect?

The effect size is the magnitude of the treatment difference as represented by the measures of association we reviewed above, whether that be an absolute risk reduction, relative risk reduction, risk ratio, hazard ratio, or odds ratio. *The confidence interval for the reported results tells you how precise the estimate of the effect size is.* The confidence interval (CI) provides more information than simply whether or not a result is statistically significant. Imagine that the same study is carried out multiple times on different patient samples. You will not get the exact same result each time. Random error dictates that there is a range within which the results will fall. The "true" result lies somewhere within the spread of results from these studies. Because each study we read is providing an estimate—called the *point estimate*—of the effect size, we ask how close it may have gotten to the "truth." The 95% confidence interval represents a statistical estimate of the range within which we will find the true effect 95% of the time (95% is usually chosen arbitrarily and sometimes you will see 99% or other confidence intervals). The confidence interval is analogous to the "neighborhood of truth." The range applies to whatever point estimate is being reported—the RR, ARR, RRR, etc. Thus, if we use this "spread" we'll theoretically only be wrong 5% of the time, or the true effect will fall outside the range 5% of the time. In other words, by convention we accept a 5% error rate—a 5% probability that this estimate occurred by chance, not by truth.

A narrower confidence interval represents less potential random error present in the results for that study. We will see below why studies with larger sample sizes tend to have narrower confidence intervals and less random error.

> *To assess the value of any confidence interval, inspect what is happening at each end. Would you be content if the true result were at either of those ends?*

What if I have a *negative study*? It is still worthwhile to inspect the confidence interval. Perhaps the interval has edged across the null point, losing statistical significance, but the majority of it lies in an area of possible treatment benefit? Perhaps the study was too small, or lacked power in another way—such as when the groups look more similar either through *contamination* (when the experimental or control group receive the intervention intended for the other arm of the study), or through loss to follow-up. The truth might be that there is still a worthwhile treatment benefit. In that situation, one would wait for larger studies or a meta-analysis of a number of smaller studies to give a more definitive answer. If the confidence interval is evenly balanced on both sides of the null point, and the study was large and had few or no methodologic flaws, then you can trust the negative, and move on. The bottom line is, look at the confidence interval in a negative study, and decide for yourself if there might be something happening at one end or the other that's worth investigating further.

The *p*-Value and How It Relates to the Confidence Interval

When a research study is initiated, the *null hypothesis* generally states that there is no difference between groups, or no effect of treatment. The *p*-value is a measure of the probability that the null hypothesis is true, or that the difference between groups occurred by chance rather than true treatment effect. If a *p*-value threshold is <0.05, it means that the probability of a *type I error* or false positive result (rejecting the null hypothesis when it was actually true) is less than 5%. While the *p*-value tells us if a result is statistically significant, the confidence interval shows us how wide the spread of possible true results was and how close they came to the edges. The confidence interval is, therefore, more informative than a p-value, on its own.

Therefore, when is the result *clinically useful*? In a positive study, one where the treatment is considered effective, one can *look at both ends of the confidence interval and ask yourself if you're comfortable if the truth were to lie at either end.* Ideally, even large trials should be repeated by other researchers and confirmed before we consider the results of one trial to be the ultimate truth.

TEACH IT!!

Therapy Math: Getting Started [15]

Visual aids to assist in teaching concepts of therapy math are also depicted in Video 4.1 which accompanies this chapter.

10 minutes:

Select a therapy study in your clinical field that finds a statistically significant difference with an intervention of interest. Working with current articles on topics that learners will actually encounter in a clinical setting tends to be well received, since they are gaining a clinical pearl while learning Therapy Math.

Consider reviewing the risk of bias of the paper first, as reviewed in prior *TEACH IT!!* tips. Then, create a 2 × 2 table on the board and work through it together as a group. Have the learners find the results table and select the outcome of interest, generally the primary outcome of the study, to populate the table. Use the 2 × 2 tables in this chapter as a guide.

Once learners have filled in the table, have them work through the Absolute Risk (i.e., event rate) in each group, and then proceed to calculate the ARR and RR by first subtracting absolute risks, and then dividing. Utilize our [Worksheets 4.1 and 4.2, Appendix] as a guide for this exercise.

Therapy Math: Absolute Risk Reduction

5–10 min:

To help visual learners grasp ARR, add visual aids such as bar graphs to demonstrate how the two event rates look side by side, with the difference between them visually apparent.

Compare the absolute risk reduction for the primary outcome in a study to the absolute risk *increase* of a *harm* noted in the study. Benefits must always be balanced with harms when approaching decision making for a patient, as well as how heavily the patient weighs those benefits vs. harms. Ask learners whether they would prescribe the intervention after weighing the potential benefits and harms.

Therapy Math: Relative Risk

5–10 min:

In EBM (and all things), a RATIO is a RATIO is a RATIO. The "Relative Risk" (RR) is synonymous with "risk ratio." In other words, it is the ratio between two event rates, one divided by the other. By convention, the risk in the intervention group goes on top and the baseline (control group) risk goes on the bottom. Thus, when the risk of an event has been reduced, the resulting risk ratio is a number less than one. When we increase the risk of an outcome, the resulting number is greater than one.

Learners sometimes confuse Relative Risk with Relative Risk Reduction—but we are not there yet! Remind them that this is just a ratio of risks. On its own, the RR is not too easy to put into words, or apply to patients.

TEACH IT!!

Therapy Math: Relative Risk Reduction [15]

15–30 min:

Now that we have calculated ARR and RR above from a sample article, move on to the Relative Risk Reduction (RRR). Distinguishing the type of information conveyed by ARR and RRR and how to use them is a core piece of EBM teaching.

We define the Relative Risk Reduction in two ways, the "numeric" way and the "intuitive" way.

Numerically, RRR = 1 − RR. Remind learners that, because the RR is a ratio, a ratio of 1 signifies the intervention or exposure had no effect. So, one way of thinking about the magnitude of the risk reduction is how far down from 1 did the ratio go? Hence, 1 − RR.

Intuitively, ask the learners how they would explain the RRR in a sentence. What does that number represent? Guide them using an explanation such as this: the RRR is telling us how much of our baseline risk has been reduced by the intervention. Specifically, the ARR is what proportion of the baseline risk? Hence, RRR = ARR/baseline risk. An analogy to help learners understand this concept is a sale in a retail store. The RRR is like the "percent-off coupon." A consumer (patient) gets a percent off (relative reduction) the full price (baseline risk) because they have a coupon (the intervention).

Calculate the RRR for the same data you used in the ARR and RR exercise above. Invariably, the RRR will be a larger number than the ARR. Talk about what that means. These numbers are just different ways to describe the SAME data! Learners should grasp that the RRR is "more impressive," and, in fact, has been shown to be more influential on decision making than the ARR.

Ask learners to imagine themselves as an industry sponsor of the trial. Which measure of effect they would use when advertising to stakeholders? Industry sponsors of randomized trials who want to maximize the impact of the findings will often focus on the RRR, because it is more impressive. Often, pharmaceutical ads will focus on the RRR and minimize the ARR.

Spend some time demonstrating the distinction between ARR and RRR. Draw a simple diagram on the board: three bar graphs showing hypothetical data such as that depicted in Fig. 4.8. Each graph has two bars, to show two event rates. For example, consider using the following event rates: 50% and 25%, 10% and 5%, 2% and 1%, and draw bars accordingly. Ask the learners to tell you the ARR for each example. The answers are 25%, 5%, and 1%. Then, ask the learners to tell you the RRR for each example. The answer is 50% in each situation. (note that the answer key matches Fig. 4.5 in the text). This visual demonstration illustrates that the *same relative risk reduction plays out very differently across different levels of baseline risk*. Also, point out that the discrepancy between RRR and ARR is greatest at the lowest event rates!! Scientific articles which report on low event rate outcomes are more likely to report only the RRR in the abstract—it takes more digging and some simple math to get the ARR.

Finally, use the three bar graphs you've drawn to make another point. What if the middle bar graph is your "data", but the first bar graph is your patient's risk? It turns out, every study contains patients with a spectrum of risk. Most studies report the average of the overall group. Using the reported result (i.e., ARR) in the study doesn't tell you how that would play out for your patient. The only thing that is *PORTABLE*, from the study, to apply to *YOUR PATIENT'S* baseline risk is the RRR (as derived from the RR). So, while it is inflated, and can be misleading, when it comes to applying results to patients, it will prove necessary. We demonstrate how to use a RRR from a study, and your patient's baseline risk of disease to calculate the patient's ARR in the chapter titled "Applying results of therapy trials to patients."

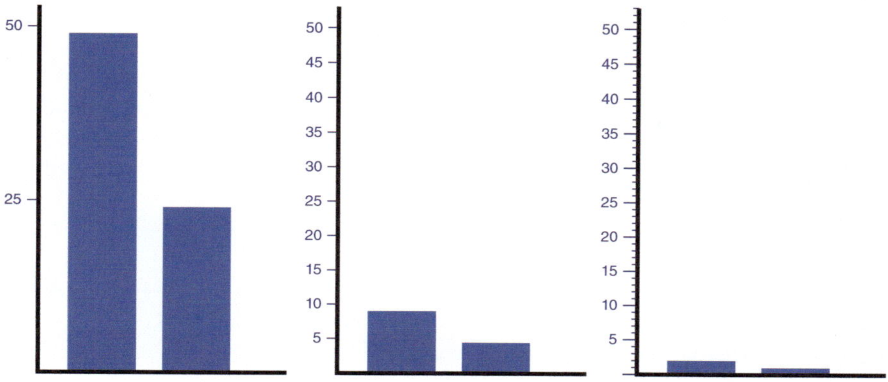

Fig. 4.8 ARR vs. RRR

TEACH IT!!

Therapy Math: Number Needed to Treat [15]

15 min:

After calculating ARR, RR, and RRR for a particular data set, ask learners if they are familiar with the Number Needed to Treat (NNT) concept. Some may not be familiar with it, and others may say, "it's 1/ARR."

Break it down by pointing out that the NNT is just a re-framing of the ARR. It is, indeed, 1/ARR. But, why?

Put up a diagram like Fig. 4.6 on the board: If the ARR is 5%, then treating 100 patients helps 5 patients avoid the outcome. Then ask, "how many people do I have to treat to help one patient?" Dividing both sides of the "equation" by 5 gives us the answer—hence, 1/ARR. Demonstrating this visually helps learners to understand how the NNT is a re-framing of the ARR.

What does the NNT mean in words? Have the learners try to use it in a sentence. Remind learners of common pitfalls to avoid when interpreting NNT:

NNT is expressed as a whole number as we cannot treat a fraction of an individual.

Furthermore, the NNT incorporates the element of time. For instance, if the NNT comes from a trial conducted over 5 years, the sentence the learners construct should include this.

Finally, point out the number of treated patients that would not benefit from the intervention. For example, if the NNT is 100, that means that for every 1 person that benefits, 99 people do not benefit from the intervention.

Compare NNTs for some common conditions, and have learners discuss [16].

Discuss the proper usage of NNT. While clinicians tend to utilize NNT as a common denominator against which to compare interventions, NNT has been shown not to be helpful with patients. In fact, the NNT does not improve patient comprehension of risk, satisfaction with the risk discussion, or decision-making ability. [12] So, proceed with caution with patients, and focus on the visually demonstrating their ARR.

Applying and Communicating Results of Clinical Trials to Your Patient

The first thing to check when deciding if a trial is relevant for your patient are the *inclusion and exclusion criteria.* These criteria indicate whether or not the investigators started with a reasonable, representative population of patients with the condition, and whether it is similar to your patient population. Based on these criteria, ask yourself if there is any compelling reason why the results should not be applied to your patient. Would your patient have been enrolled? If so, great. If not, why not? Is your patient more sick than the study group, or less? Sometimes, if your patient is slightly outside the bounds of the inclusion criteria, you may still opt to utilize the data as a ballpark estimate, if no other relevant data exists. Consider demographic factors such as age, race, and gender, clinical factors such as disease stage or type, and social context. Were the study population's resources similar to your patient, in terms of economic status, education level, insurance status, access to care, environment, and culture?

If you decide that the study results are relevant to your patient, the next step is to assess how the magnitude of effect will impact your patient. We will consider your own patient's risk of disease, as compared to the average study participant, and then apply the reduction in risk to your patient's starting point.

Case Scenario

You are seeing a patient in the primary care clinic who is transferring her care from out of state. She is a 63-year-old Caucasian woman with hypertension, hyperlipidemia, and tobacco use. Her health maintenance is up to date. She is 5′ 7″ and weighs 135 lbs. She has the results of a bone densitometry done 1 year ago, with T scores in the range of −2.1 at the femoral neck. She states that her previous physician said this was an adequate score and she need not be concerned with therapy for osteoporosis. She is still a little nervous though, because her mother had a hip fracture at age 78. Do you need to perform additional testing? Do you need to prescribe calcium and vitamin D? Is she a candidate for bisphosphonate therapy? You are not sure how her family history affects her personal risk of fracture.

Think about this case as you read about the concepts below, and we will resolve the case shortly.

Estimating the Patient-Specific Risk Reduction

What is the patient's chance of benefiting from treatment? What we need is to know our patient's *baseline risk* of an outcome, and then data to assess *how much that risk will change with the intervention.* If the study population does not exactly reflect your patient's characteristics, then you cannot simply apply the ARR from the study to your patient, because the baseline risk will differ. Remember that even within a study, there is a spectrum of risk, and the average risk in the study is generally what is reported. This average risk may not reflect your patient's risk. Therefore, to apply results from the study to your patient, we use the one metric that's portable—remember, that's one positive quality of the RRR! *We apply the RRR from the study to OUR patient's baseline risk to get OUR patient's ARR.* See below.

Let us remember some of the basic math from the Therapy Math section:

> ARR (absolute risk reduction) = "Subtract" absolute risks.
> RRR (relative risk reduction) = ARR/baseline risk.
> Therefore, ARR = RRR × baseline risk.

We will use the formula to apply a RRR to our patient to get the ARR for our patient, *ARR = [RRR × baseline risk].* See the resolution of the bone density case below.

This change in the baseline risk can also be calculated for harmful interventions, and we refer to the *RRI, or relative risk increase*, instead of RRR. The corresponding ARI, or absolute risk increase, is calculated in similar fashion to ARR. *ARI = [RRI × baseline risk].*

Deciding on your patient's baseline risk is challenging, and can be drawn from your clinical judgment, published data from cohorts or randomized trials, the epidemiology sections of medical reference resources, and/or clinical prediction rules.

Resolution of our Case

Now we know that in order to come to our own patient's ARR for benefit from an intervention, *we need to know two things: (1) her baseline risk of fracture and (2) the relative risk reduction associated with the intervention.*

Where can we get information on her baseline risk of fracture? If you checked in a clinical database first, you would quickly learn that the World Health Organization has created a fracture risk assessment tool, called FRAX, available online. If you use this tool, you find she has a 10-year risk of hip fracture of 1.7%. Can we improve on this? By how much?

Where can we get information on the relative risk reduction associated with, say, bisphosphonate therapy? You suspect there are multiple trials on this topic, so you look for a Cochrane systematic review on your library website. You put "bisphosphonate" in the search field, and the first relevant citation you see is a review of alendronate for primary and secondary reduction in fracture risk. You find there is an overall relative risk reduction for hip fracture of 50% using alendronate. Now we have enough information, so let us do the math:

ARR = RRR × baseline risk = (0.50 × 0.017) = 0.0085, or 0.85%. In other words, her fracture risk would go from 1.7% over 10 years to 0.85% over 10 years if she took a bisphosphonate.

What do you think of that? There are some known side effects to bisphosphonates, so you may hold off for now. The benefits are probably not worth the cost and the hassle. (it turns out, a threshold of 3% for the 10-year risk of hip fracture is recommended by experts as a starting point for bisphosphonates).

How Should Results Be Communicated to the Patient?

We have calculated OUR patient's baseline risk of fracture, gleaned the RRR from a study, and calculated our patient's absolute risk reduction with bisphosphonates. Which numerical format should we use to convey this to the patient in order to maximize her comprehension of the risk and benefit and comfort with making a decision, thereby improving the likelihood of her deciding to take a medicine for her bones?

A systematic review of methods of communicating probabilities to patients concluded that the following principles should be used: Use absolute risks, not relative risks, and visually demonstrate the baseline risk and risk reduction with a visual aid, such as a bar graph or an icon array [12]. It turns out that using the NNT with patients is NOT helpful. Multiple studies found NNT inferior when it comes to patients' comprehension and decision-making ability.

Some resources are publicly available to assist in the process of visually displaying baseline risks and how treatments improve that risk. For examples, explore the following websites:

Use of bisphosphonates in the treatment of osteoporosis:
https://osteoporosisdecisionaid.mayoclinic.org
Use of statins in the primary prevention of cardiovascular disease:
https://statindecisionaid.mayoclinic.org/

Another option is to create your own icon array, for risk reductions of interventions you discuss routinely with patients. Consider creating your own using publicly available tools created at the University of Michigan:
http://www.iconarray.com/

What if My Patient Has Only Been Studied as a *Subgroup* of a Trial?

Are the authors listing valuable differences between patients with different underlying risks, or are they simply "data-dredging" to come up with results that appear interesting? Understanding subgroup analyses begins with attention to the measures of effect that are reported. While the RRR reduction may be very similar across different subgroups, the ARR will often vary widely due to differences in baseline risk. It is important to remember that even among subjects within a study there exists a spectrum of baseline risk. Subgroups are one illustration of that variability.

Remember that a subgroup analysis may not give an accurate estimate of the effect of the intervention because the subgroup was not randomized, in and of itself [17]. You may have uneven numbers in the experimental groups, or uneven rates of comorbidities. One way for researchers to avoid this problem is to *stratify* their randomization up front by variables that they anticipate will have an impact on their results. If a study is stratified by a particular variable, meaning those with and without the variable are randomized, then looking at that variable as a sub-group later is more reliable. For example, a study of a cardiovascular drug may stratify by diabetes status, ensuring that their concealed randomization process will spread diabetic patients evenly across the two groups. They anticipate that diabetes will affect cardiovascular outcomes. Later, looking at diabetics as a subgroup is more reliable, because it IS a randomized comparison.

Remember also that a subgroup is just that, a *smaller* part of the group. Because it is a smaller group, it is more subject to random error. Any conclusions made about a subgroup in one trial should ideally be confirmed by other trials focused on that group. The statistical tests involved in subgroup analyses should have stringent thresholds and account for a random error associated with making multiple comparisons [18].

Because of the limitations of a subgroup analysis, we should expect at the minimum that authors will specify their planned subgroup analyses *a priori*, and *limit the overall number*. Subgroups that are designated after a study is finished may be more subject to bias on the part of the investigators, as results may drive their curiosity about certain questions, but not others. The greater the number of subgroups examined, the greater the tendency to find differences by chance alone as the sheer volume of comparisons increases. Subgroup findings should make clinical sense, and ideally should be replicated in other studies.

TEACH IT!!

Applying Results of Therapy Trials to Patients: Calculating the Individual Absolute Risk Reduction

30 min:

This session can directly follow the session covering ARR, RR, and RRR above. If it stands alone in the future after teaching ARR, RR, and RRR, it should first briefly refresh learners' memory of those concepts. Worksheet 4.3, in the appendix, can serve as an example.

Remind learners that RRR = ARR/Baseline Risk. If we know the RRR from a reliable RCT or meta-analysis and we can calculate or estimate our patient's baseline risk for the outcome, then we can solve for *our patient's absolute risk reduction* and our patient's number needed to treat.

The clinical example of statin therapy for primary prevention of cardiovascular disease in adults works well, because there are Cochrane systematic reviews providing estimates of the RRR and there is a widely used atherosclerotic cardiovascular disease (ASCVD) risk estimator to establish your patient's baseline risk of cardiovascular events, which can be found at: http://tools.acc.org/ASCVD-Risk-Estimator-Plus/#!/calculate/estimate/.

Have learners read through the abstract you provide to extract the most relevant RRR.

Have learners calculate the baseline risk for a sample patient you provide.

Have learners do the math to solve for ARR, and then NNT. How would they explain the results of these calculations in words to a colleague? How would they communicate the same information to a patient? Discuss the importance of adding visual aids such as bar graphs or icon arrays to demonstrate the data.

The statin example is also ideal because of the Mayo Clinic Statin Decision Aid, which can be found at: https://statindecisionaid.mayoclinic.org/. Once the learners have done the math for themselves, pull up the decision aid online and review together. This decision aid instantly creates two icon arrays, one for the baseline risk of cardiovascular disease, and one for the incremental benefit of adding a statin. Play with the risk calculator a bit to demonstrate how things change clinically when a patient is a smoker vs. non-smoker, older vs. younger. The American Heart Association and the American College of Cardiology have set a recommended threshold of 7.5% ten-year risk of cardiovascular disease as a place to start a statin. Do your learners agree that this is a good starting place? Some may, some may not. They are ALL correct! Ultimately, this is the patient's decision. Our job as clinicians is to provide the information in a format that facilitates patient understanding and discuss risks and benefits as we understand them. Patients are then able to make their own informed choice.

Shared Decision Making

Another key piece of applying results to patients is the patient's entire context of care. In fact, none of this evidence even matters if we cannot effectively communicate these concepts to patients and improve not only their understanding of the decision before them, but their comfort in making that decision. *Shared decision making (SDM)* is defined as "*a collaborative process that allows patients and their providers to make health care decisions together, taking into account the best scientific evidence available, as well as the patient's values and preferences*" [19]. As you have guessed by now, knowing and understanding the evidence is just the first step—the next step is about making it accessible to patients in real time in the clinical context. We address this topic more fully in the chapter entitled Shared Decision Making.

Appendix: Worksheets

Worksheet 4.0: Critical Appraisal for a Therapy Study

Therapy Critical Appraisal Worksheet (Randomized Controlled Trials)

Assessing the risk of bias	
Was randomization carried out, via objective, computerized process?	
Was the allocation of subjects to randomly determined groups concealed?	
Did the intervention and control groups subsequently have similar proportions of prognostic variables?	
Were subjects, investigators, statisticians, and outcome adjudicators blinded to treatment group?	
Were the study groups treated equally, aside from the intervention of interest?	
Was follow-up as complete as can be reasonably expected?	
Was an intention-to-treat analysis performed?	
If the trial was stopped early, did investigators adhere to a pre-specified stopping threshold while maintaining statistical rigor?	
Assessing the results	
What is the magnitude and precision of the results?	
Can the results be applied to my patient population?	

Worksheet 4.1: Therapy Exercise, Blank Sample

Therapy Worksheet

The Case: [Create a case describing a patient with a therapy dilemma connected to the teaching article you have chosen to use. For teaching purposes, choosing the article first and fashioning the case to match allows you to focus on the features of the article that you want to convey to the learners.]

Question 1: Assess the risk of bias of the paper you have chosen

Calculations: Construct the following 2 × 2 table, and perform the calculations below. Where do you find the information to fill out the table?

	Outcome	No Outcome
Exposure		
Control		

Absolute Risk of Outcome with Exposure: ____________

Absolute Risk of Outcome with Control: ________________

ARR ("subtract") = _________________________

RR ("divide") = __________________________

RRR = __________________________________

NNT = __________________________________

Advanced concepts to consider: [this will vary with the paper you select]

- Composite outcomes—what are the pieces of the composite? Which occurred most frequently, or drove the results? How do we apply that clinically?
- Secondary outcomes—generally considered "hypothesis generating."
- Power.
- Statistical significance vs. clinical significance.
- Kaplan–Meier curves.

Worksheet 4.2: Therapy Exercise, Internal Medicine Sample

Therapy Worksheet: Internal Medicine Sample

The Case: A 60-year-old man with hypertension, tobacco abuse, and a history of MI 8 years ago presents to the clinic for routine follow-up. His blood pressure and lipids are well controlled on lisinopril 10 qd, carvedilol 6.25 bid, and atorvastatin 80 qd. His LDL is 85. He has been reading about new agents for preventing heart attacks, PCSK-9 inhibitors, and wonders if he should try them.

Question 1: Using the User's Guide criteria summarized in your handout, assess the risk of bias of the FOURIER trial of Evolocumab, from the New England Journal of Medicine, May 2017.

Calculations: Construct the following 2 × 2 table, and perform the calculations below. Where do you find the information to fill out the table?

	Outcome	No Outcome
Exposure		
Control		

Absolute Risk of CVD composite with Evolocumab: ____________

Absolute Risk of CVD composite with Placebo: ______________

ARR ("subtract") = ______________________

RR ("divide") = _________________________

RRR = ______________________________

NNT = ______________________________

Concepts to review with this paper:

- Composite outcomes—what are the pieces of the composite? Which occurred most frequently, or drove the results? How do we apply that clinically?
- Secondary outcomes—generally considered "hypothesis generating."
- Kaplan–Meier curves.

Worksheet 4.3: Applying Results Exercise, Internal Medicine Sample

Applying Results to Patients Worksheet: Internal Medicine

[We provide this example to demonstrate an instance where the following criteria are met: (1) A calculator for baseline risk of CVD events exists, (2) Data on relative risk reduction exists, (3) The condition is encountered commonly in clinical settings, and (4) the findings can be contrasted with another agent for the same condition]

The Case: You are seeing a 55-year-old Caucasian man in clinic for an annual exam. He has no complaints. You are following him for hypertension only. He takes chlorthalidone. Recent blood work has been normal, he does not smoke, and he is up to date with a colonoscopy. At this visit, when reviewing family history, he reminds you that his father died of a heart attack in his mid-fifties, and he has been wondering if there is anything else he can do to prevent heart attacks or other vascular events.

Today's blood pressure is 142/80.
Lipid panel shows: Tot Chol 212, Trig 154, HDL 35, LDL 128

Remember, an individual patient's *ARR = (RRR × baseline risk)*

1. Where do you find information on his baseline risk of MI or cardiovascular events? Calculate his baseline risk.

2. Where do you find information about the relative risk reduction in cardiovascular curevents with statins? Calculate your patient's ARR and NNT.

3. How about your patient's ARR and NNT with aspirin?

4. Can you assess the number needed to harm for GI bleed with aspirin?

References

1. Higgins JPT, Green S, Cochrane Collaboration. Section 8, "Assessing risk of bias in included studies". In: Higgins JPT, Green S, editors. Cochrane handbook for systematic reviews of interventions version 5.0.0. London: Cochrane Collaboration; 2008.
2. Schulz KF, et al. Empirical evidence of bias: dimensions of methodological quality associated with estimates of treatment effects in controlled trials. JAMA. 1995;273(5):408–12.
3. Schulz KF, Grimes DA. Generation of allocation sequences in randomized trials: chance, not choice. Lancet. 2002;359:515–9.
4. Montori VA, Jaeschke R, et al. Users' guides to detecting misleading claims in clinical research reports. BMJ. 2004;329:1093–6.
5. Gralnek IM, Dulai GS, et al. Esomeprazole vs other proton pump inhibitors in erosive esophagitis: a meta-analysis of randomized clinical trials. Clin Gastroenterol Hepatol. 2006;4(12):1452–8.
6. Montori VM, Guyatt GH. Intention-to-treat principle. CMAJ. 2001;165(10):1339–41.
7. Bassler D, Briel M, et al. Stopping randomized trials early for benefit and estimation of treatment effects: systematic review and meta-regression analysis. JAMA. 2010;303(12):1180–7.
8. Montori VM, Devereaux PJ, et al. Randomized trials stopped early for benefit: a systematic review. JAMA. 2005;294:2203–9.
9. Ioannidis JPA. Why most published research findings are false. PLoS Med. 2005;2(8):e124.
10. Alhazzani W, Walter SD, Jaeschke R, Cook DJ, Guyatt G. Does treatment lower risk? Understanding the results. In: Users' guides to the medical literature: a manual for evidence-based clinical practice. 3rd ed. Chicago: American Medical Association; 2008.
11. Laupacis A, Sackett DL, Roberts RS. An assessment of clinically useful measures of the consequences of treatment. N Engl J Med. 1988;318(26):1728–33.
12. Zipkin DA, Umscheid CA, et al. Evidence-based risk communication: a systematic review. Ann Intern Med. 2014;161:270–80.
13. Rochwerg B, Elbarbary M, Jaeschke R, Walter SD, Guyatt G. Understanding the results: more about odds ratios. In: Users' guides to the medical literature: a manual for evidence-based clinical practice. 3rd ed. Chicago: American Medical Association; 2015.
14. Spruance SL, Reid JE, et al. Hazard ratio in clinical trials. Antimicrob Agents Chemother. 2004;48:2787–92.
15. Barratt A, Wyer PC, et al. Tips for learners of evidence-based medicine: 1. Relative risk reduction, absolute risk reduction, and number needed to treat. CMAJ. 2004;171(4):353–8.
16. Urrutia G, Ferreira-Gonzalez I, Guyatt G, Devereaux PJ. Numbers needed to treat. In: Users' guides to the medical literature: a manual for evidence-based clinical practice. 3rd ed. Chicago: American Medical Association; 2015.
17. Higgins JPT, Green S, Cochrane Collaboration. Section 9.6.2, "What are subgroup analyses?". In: Higgins JPT, Green S, editors. Cochrane handbook for systematic reviews of interventions version 5.0.0. London: Cochrane Collaboration; 2008.
18. Wang R, Lagakos SW, et al. Statistics in medicine—reporting of subgroup analyses in clinical trials. N Engl J Med. 2007;357:21.
19. Informed Medical Decisions Foundation. https://innovations.ahrq.gov/qualitytools/informed-medical-decisions-foundation-tools-providers. Accessed 2 Jan 2019.

Non-inferiority Study Designs

5

Daniella A. Zipkin and Matthew Tuck

Guide for the Teacher

Non-inferiority trial designs have emerged as an increasingly common design over the years in parallel with the increase in studies of comparative effectiveness of two active interventions. The topic of non-inferiority was incorporated into the Users' Guides to the Medical Literature for the first time in 2015, following several papers written about their strengths and weaknesses [1, 2]. Because non-inferiority designs are also randomized controlled trials, their special features and pitfalls are frequently missed by clinicians and academics alike. In addition, a far higher proportion of non-inferiority trials actually conclude non-inferiority than traditional superiority designs conclude superiority. In other words, it is easier to find non-inferiority, because all of the forces that work to lower a study's power make it MORE likely that non-inferiority will be found. For this reason, we feel is it incredibly important that EBM learners have a sense of features of non-inferiority trials which distinguish them from

Supplementary Information The online version contains supplementary material available at [https://doi.org/10.1007/978-3-031-11174-7_5].

D. A. Zipkin (✉)
Department of Medicine, Duke University Health System,
Duke University School of Medicine, Durham, NC, USA
e-mail: daniella.zipkin@duke.edu

M. Tuck
Department of Medicine, Veterans Affairs Medical Center, Medical Service,
George Washington University, Washington, DC, USA
e-mail: Matthew.Tuck@va.gov

D. A. Zipkin (ed.), *Teaching Evidence-Based Medicine*,
https://doi.org/10.1007/978-3-031-11174-7_5

traditional superiority trials, and keep a critical eye towards sources of bias and lack of power.

Because non-inferiority is a relatively new topic, there may not be many faculty available who feel comfortable teaching it. It is our hope that with the detailed descriptions and videos that follow, faculty who are teaching therapy will be able to easily transition to adding non-inferiority.

We recommend allotting at least 1 hour to the topic as a standalone teaching session, and we encourage reiterating these concepts in any case conference or journal club where the non-inferiority design comes up. Non-inferiority must follow Therapy—learners must have a good grasp of randomized controlled trials in general, and the sources of bias within them.

The core topics to cover in non-inferiority designs include:

What is a non-inferiority design?
What is the non-inferiority margin and how is it derived?
What are the key sources of bias in non-inferiority trials?
How does the power calculation differ in non-inferiority trials?

Non-inferiority Study Designs

To get a new drug on the market, the United States Food and Drug Administration (FDA) historically required the drug manufacturer to prove efficacy over placebo. They didn't necessarily demand "comparative effectiveness" with active treatments. However, once superiority over placebo has been clearly demonstrated for a drug class, if the condition carries significant morbidity when untreated, then randomizing patients to placebo is no longer ethical [1]. When a new drug class is developed and adds appealing features the current option does not have, such as ease of administration or less monitoring, it may only need to be "as good as" current therapies. Or, perhaps, simply "not worse than" current therapies. In that case, being "not worse than" the first line therapy would still confer some additional benefits. Take, for example, the case of anticoagulation for atrial fibrillation to prevent stroke. Warfarin has clearly established efficacy over placebo in the past. When the oral factor Xa inhibitor drugs were developed for prevention of thromboembolism, they offered the advantage of not needing repetitive INR testing. If they are not worse than warfarin, they may be perceived as an improvement over warfarin. Therefore, the non-inferiority trial design may be an appropriate way to test them.

Non-inferiority is a modern design with interesting features and a whole host of statistical and methodological concepts making them unique from traditional trials. They emerged as a chapter in the Users' Guides to the Medical Literature for the first time in 2015 [2, 3]. Here, we will run through the key concepts in understanding these special trials.

The Non-inferiority Margin: Just How Much "Worse" Can You Be and Still Be Considered "Not Worse Than"?

Non-inferiority margins represent the boundary of how much "worse" a new intervention can be compared to the existing one, and still be considered non-inferior. The margin should be chosen based on historical trials of the original intervention's comparison to placebo. Some portion of that historical benefit must be preserved. It can be stated in *absolute terms*, such as an actual acceptable absolute difference in risk, or in *relative terms*, such as the proportion of prior benefit that must be preserved.

The FDA has suggested the following guideline for choosing a non-inferiority margin [1]: Start with the smallest plausible benefit of the existing active treatment. This means the "most conservative" edge of the *confidence interval* of the prior superiority of active treatment vs. placebo or prior comparator (the edge of the confidence interval closest to no effect). Then, your margin should maintain some proportion of that historical benefit. By convention, this is typically 50% of the prior margin of benefit. We demonstrate this visually in the video tutorials which accompany this chapter.

While many investigators follow the FDA's recommended method for calculating a non-inferiority margin, some do not. Margins may be calculated based on expert consensus, or even arbitrarily, when no baseline data are available to inform the decision. Here is the catch: remember what we learned about *random error* and smaller differences in event rates? The *TIGHTER* the non-inferiority margin, the *MORE* patients need to be recruited to maintain the power to find that difference. Conversely, the *LARGER* the non-inferiority margin, the *FEWER* patients need to be recruited. Because *in non-inferiority trials investigators are looking for no difference*, it is actually in their interests to widen the non-inferiority margin. Widening the margin makes it less expensive to run the study, and easier to find non-inferiority. However, the wider the margin, the less clinical significance we can apply to the finding of non-inferiority. *There is an inherent conflict of interest for the investigators when selecting their non-inferiority margin.* Perhaps we should have separate adjudication committees selecting the margins, to guard against this form of bias being built into the study framework.

There are also some assumptions that go into selecting the margin. If you are working to establish that your new therapy is not inferior to an older therapy, then that older therapy must still perform well now. Therapies that may not stand the test of time include anti-microbials, because of shifts in resistance over time, and anti-neoplastic agents, because of advances in the field of oncology, for instance. See Box 5.1:

Box 5.1 Non-inferiority Assumptions [4]

Assay sensitivity: active control would have been superior to placebo if placebo were used.

Constancy: the historical difference between active control and placebo is assumed to hold now.

Variability: if estimates of historical benefit over placebo vary, use the smallest (some debate here).

What Are the Results and How Do We Interpret Them?

Non-inferiority studies first ask the statistical question of non-inferiority, which is a one-directional or one-tailed test. (This differs from "equivalence," where the deviation could go in either direction, and is a two-tailed test). They have the option, if non-inferiority is met, to then ask the question of superiority from the same data. This is like "spending" the other statistical tail on superiority. It is a bit like coming to the conclusion of superiority through the back door, since you didn't recruit as many subjects at the outset as you would have if you had designed the study as superiority from the beginning. Figure 5.1 illustrates potential findings that can occur.

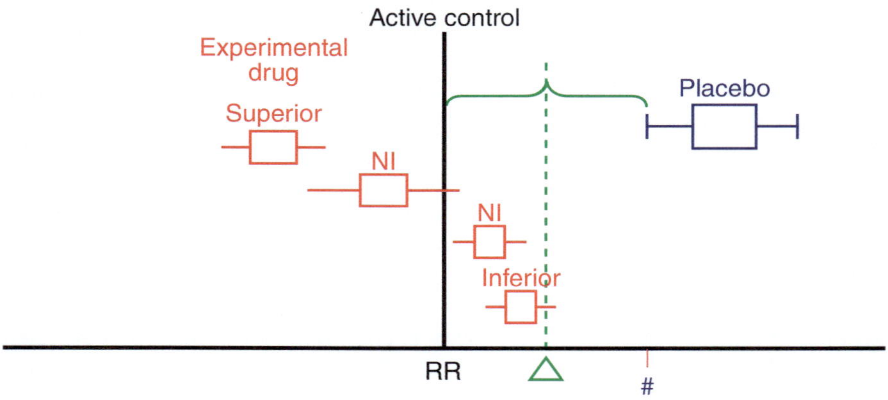

Fig. 5.1 Potential results from a non-inferiority study. Red squares indicate summary relative risk, horizontal lines indicate confidence intervals. As long as the confidence interval does not touch the non-inferiority margin, non-inferiority is met. *NI* = non-inferior

Risk of Bias in Non-inferiority Studies

Remember all of those important methodologic steps for randomized controlled trials, designed to make sure that both groups are completely equal with regard to everything except the intervention? Well, maintaining equal chance for the outcome in both groups throughout the study, through good randomization, equal treatment, blinding, complete follow-up, and intention to treat, all serve to make it *harder* to find a difference between the groups, so that, in a traditional superiority trial, if a difference is found you can be confident that it is due to the intervention. Now, non-inferiority studies are *trying* to find *no difference. As it happens, all of those validity criteria make it easier for a non-inferiority study to conclude non-inferiority. Traditional validity criteria, while still important in any scientific experiment, don't protect us from bias as much as they do with superiority designs.*

Before you discard the risk of bias criteria, remember that we still need those protections from bias. We simply need to approach them differently, with a more critical eye. *Anything that compromises the ability to find a difference between groups if one is really there, will make a conclusion of non-inferiority less valid* [5]. We can still do a few things to protect ourselves from bias, despite this dilemma. See the next Box 5.2.

Box 5.2 Managing Bias in Non-inferiority Studies [5]

Plan the *power* calculation stringently.

Account for drop-outs stringently.

Use more than one outcome assessor, to avoid loss of power do to under-cataloguing outcome events.

Add a "per protocol" analysis to your intention to treat analysis? See below.

Using more than one outcome assessor may not be immediately intuitive. Imagine for a moment that the outcome assessor, the person determining if a clinical event meets the criteria for an outcome set forward by the investigators, is TRULY completely blinded to group assignment. If that person has a bias towards one intervention, can they exert that bias on their interpretation of outcome events? They cannot! Now imagine that the same outcome assessor believes there is truly no difference between the interventions. Can they exert that bias on the data, even if fully blinded? In fact, they can. By simply "under calling" all of the outcomes, regardless of group assignment, the study may lack the power it set out to have. For this reason, we suggest using more than one outcome assessor, and evaluating their level of agreement.

More About Power in Non-inferiority Designs

As a review, in a standard superiority design, power represents the probability of finding a difference if one is really there, or the probability of avoiding a type II error (false negative trial). In superiority designs, the null hypothesis is that there is no difference, while the alternative hypothesis is that there is a difference. This is FLIPPED around in non-inferiority designs [6]. In non-inferiority designs, the null hypothesis is that there is a difference in favor of standard treatment. The alternative hypothesis, which we are seeking to find, is that the experimental treatment is better than or only slightly worse than the standard treatment, within the margin that was defined. Therefore, power in a non-inferiority study represents the probability that non-inferiority is true, or "the power to find non-inferiority." When a non-inferiority study does not maintain the power it set out to achieve, for instance if fewer outcomes emerge than were expected, then non-inferiority becomes harder to find. With fewer events, greater random error, and therefore wider confidence intervals around the effect estimate, it is harder for those confidence intervals to stay within the pre-specified margin. Therefore, if power is compromised, but non-inferiority is still found despite that, examine the event rates carefully, and ask yourself if you are comfortable with the conclusion of non-inferiority at either end of the confidence interval. And, of course, if power is compromised and a study fails to find non-inferiority, it is at risk of having missed true non-inferiority.

That Pesky "Per-protocol Analysis"

No one in the EBM community is very comfortable with breaching the sanctity of intention-to-treat analysis. However, in non-inferiority designs, taking a look at how the per-protocol analysis plays out can serve as a sanity check for your intention-to-treat findings [5]. Here is how this works: If the intention-to-treat analysis finds no difference between groups, but the per-protocol analysis DOES find a difference, we must question whether non-inferiority is valid. It is possible that the finding of non-inferiority resulted from diluting both groups with the results of participants whose outcomes are not really known. Figure 5.2 provides a schematic diagram to help explain. In the scenario below, you can see that the intention-to-treat analysis would miss a difference by dilution of an outcome differential between the groups. When we include all participants, even those who we could not follow-up for all potential outcomes, a true difference between the groups may be lost. Keep in mind that the same does NOT apply in reverse. If a difference IS found in the intention-to-treat analysis, the analysis should stop there. Adding a per-protocol analysis after that may show no difference simply due to the loss of power as fewer subjects are analyzed.

In Box 5.3 below we summarize the discussion of features of non-inferiority trials which impact bias.

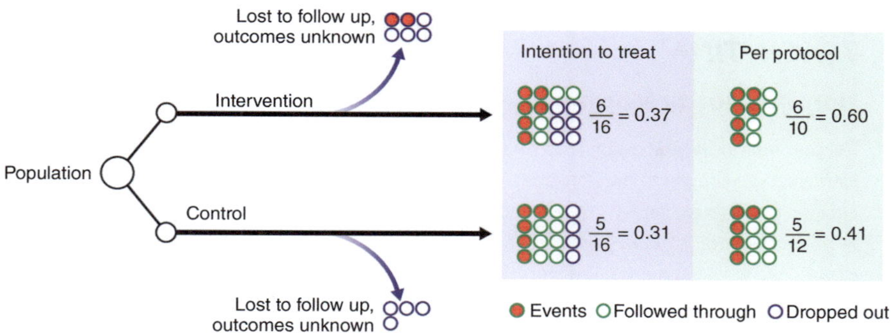

Fig. 5.2 Adding a per-protocol analysis to your intention-to-treat analysis. In some cases, adding a per-protocol analysis can uncover a difference that is missed by the intention to treat analysis, as illustrated in this hypothetical example. Notice that when we count those lost to follow-up, without knowing whether or not they had the outcome event, we dilute the denominator and may miss a real effect. The per protocol analysis, in this case removing those lost to follow-up, reveals a potential real difference

Box 5.3 Summary of Key Features of Non-Inferiority Trials Related to Potential Bias

- Was the non-inferiority margin developed based on prior placebo-controlled studies, using the most conservative estimate of the benefit over placebo? Did the margin make clinical sense?
- Was power defined a priori, rigorous, and maintained throughout the study by complete follow-up and reaching the expected number of outcome events?
- Did the methods adhere to good practices regarding randomized controlled trials (please see Chap. 4 for full details), including:
  - Randomized.
  - Concealed allocation of the randomization scheme.
  - Blinding of participants, investigators, outcome adjudicators, and data managers; Utilizing more than one outcome assessor and ensuring agreement.
  - Equal treatment of both groups.
  - Complete follow-up, with any drop outs accounted for.
  - Analysis by intention to treat, with the option of adding a per-protocol analysis.
- Was assay sensitivity preserved: Was the active control treatment administered well and would prior benefit over placebo still hold today? Check the event rates in the current trial compared to historical trials. Higher event rates may mean the active control was sub-optimal, or may signal differences in the populations studied.
- Was a "per protocol" analysis added to the intention-to-treat analysis? If results are similar to intention-to-treat results, a conclusion of non-inferiority is more reliable.

TEACH IT!!

Non-inferiority Margin

For non-inferiority studies, once the main comparison is known, we recommended teaching learners to go straight to the statistics section to see how the non-inferiority margin was calculated. Emphasize that we can use our own clinical judgment to decide if the margin is set at a point where, if the new intervention has an event rate that pushes to the edge of that margin, we would agree that it is still clinically non-inferior. There is no standard practice for calculating a non-inferiority margin. They can be generated from either relative differences or absolute difference. Margins should be calculated with this in mind: we aim to preserve some proportion of the historical benefit of the active intervention vs placebo. We recommend teaching the approach of calculating the margin to preserve at least 50% of the relative benefit of active drug vs placebo, when several prior trials of active drug vs placebo are available to provide a stable estimate of that earlier effect. This is emerging as the standard acceptable method. In this example, our figures utilize the data from the ARISTOTLE trial of Apixaban vs Warfarin for preventing stroke in atrial fibrillation, as its methodology was good [7].

The teaching tools described here are also depicted in Video 5.1 *which accompanies this chapter.*

15–30 min:

Start with a general schematic to illustrate the concept of the non-inferiority (NI) margin. Put (Fig. 5.3) on the board, sequentially adding placebo, then drug A, then new drug B, in contrasting colors. Indicate the margin, as in Fig. 5.4 and pose to the group a philosophical dilemma: "How much worse than drug A can drug B and still be considered not-worse-than drug A?"

Another good question to ask the group regarding the margin is, "what would happen to the required sample size if we made the NI margin narrower, such the two drugs had to be closer in their event rates in order to be considered non-inferior?". Based on the principles of random error, we would have to recruit MORE patients to conclude non-inferiority, if we narrow the NI margin. In other words, the more clinically rigorous the margin is, the harder it is to fund and conduct the study. This creates an inherent conflict of interest. Have the group discuss. Would it be useful to have adjudication committees for the purpose of vetting the margins? Perhaps.

Now, transition to demonstrating how a margin can be calculated, starting with (Fig. 5.5), a simple forest plot depicting the prior benefit of active drug A vs placebo, with drug A on the left side. Then, tell the group it's helpful to reframe this effect size as how much WORSE placebo was than drug A—drawing (Fig. 5.6) and flipping the effect size marker over to the right side and labeling it as placebo. In this forest plot, the "line of no difference" can now be labeled "drug A". Draw a bracket that connects the line of no difference and the closest end of the confidence interval for placebo's effect. This is the historic difference between active drug and placebo. If we wish to preserve at least 50% of that, then we will bisect it with a vertical dotted line in a contrasting color, halfway through that distance as shown in Fig. 5.7. This vertical line is the NI margin.

You can add to the diagram to indicate several possible outcomes, as shown in Fig. 5.8. Have the group discuss what each of these scenarios represents. Options range from superiority, to non-inferiority, to inferiority, as well as indeterminate, as indicated in Fig. 5.1. Non-inferiority is maintained as long as the confidence interval of the current effect estimate does not touch the NI margin.

Add other examples from the literature in your field for learners to use as you teach this session. We recommend comparing and contrasting at least two papers in order to teach this session.

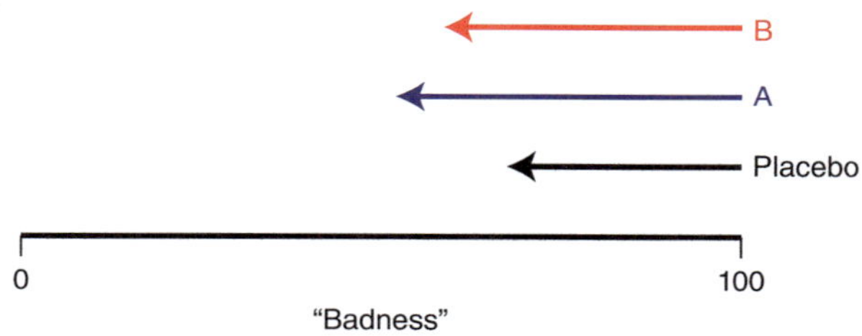

Fig. 5.3 Non-inferiority schematic

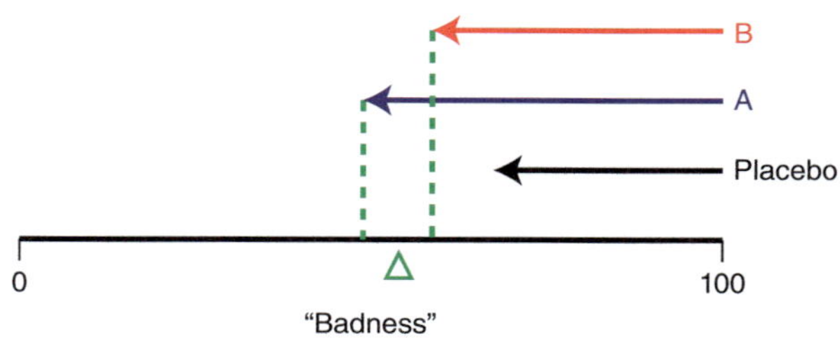

Fig. 5.4 Non-inferiority margin schematic

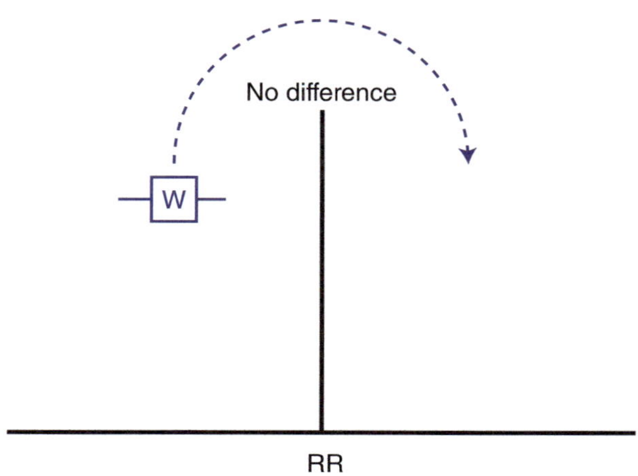

Fig. 5.5 Non-inferiority margin derivation 1. *W* = warfarin

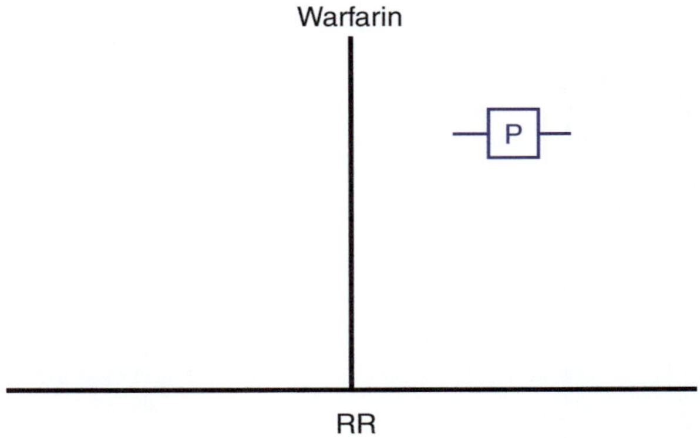

Fig. 5.6 Non-inferiority margin derivation 2. *P* = placebo

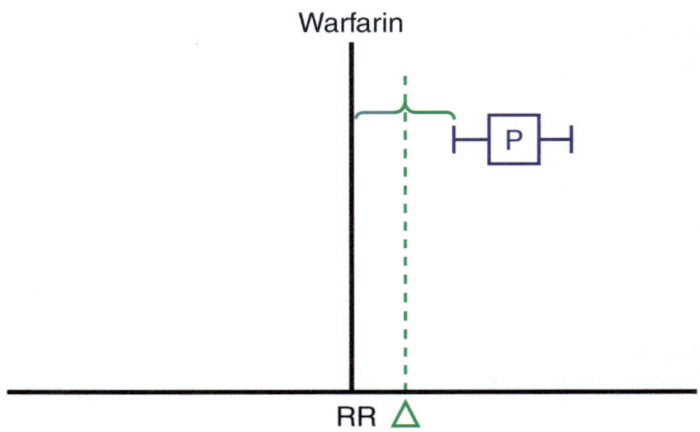

Fig. 5.7 Non-inferiority margin derivation 3. *P* = placebo

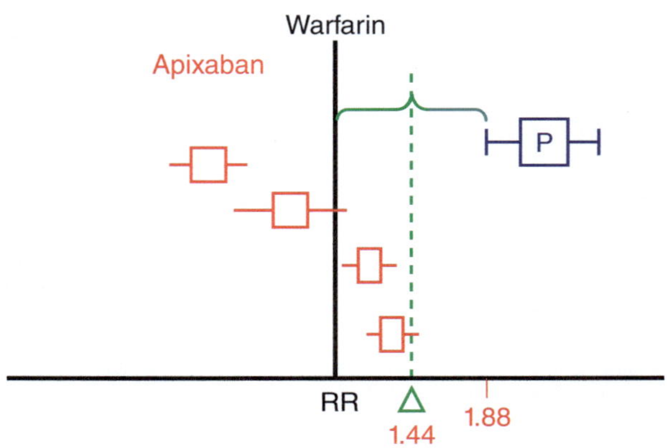

Fig. 5.8 Non-inferiority trials, possible outcomes. *P* = placebo

Bias in Non-inferiority Trials

This section must follow a session on Therapy, including sources of bias in randomized controlled trials. This section assumes learners already have a grasp of the importance of randomization, allocation concealment, blinding, equal treatment, complete follow-up, and intention-to-treat. We recommend moving through these points as a discussion amongst the learners, ideally in reference to sample articles you have shared with them. Use the Non-inferiority Critical Appraisal Worksheet, Worksheet 5.0, in the Appendix as a reference.

15 min:

Review the sources of bias in traditional superiority designs with your learners. Remind them of the key features, which are randomization, allocation concealment, blinding, equal treatment, complete follow-up, and intention-to-treat, and then ask them why these are important. What is the overall goal? The answer they should come to should be along the lines of minimizing bias, spreading confounding variables evenly between the groups, and keeping the groups as equal as possible so that, at the end of the study, you can be sure that the intervention was driving the difference seen.

Now ask the group, if all of those features are intended to keep the groups equal, making it HARDER to find a difference between them, what happens when the design is non-inferiority? ALL OF THOSE FEATURES, WHEN DONE WELL, MAKE IT EASIER TO CONCLUDE NON-INFERIORITY. This is a big deal! The features that make an RCT a reliable scientific experiment do NOT protect us from erroneously concluding non-inferiority. So, what do we do? We cannot simply abandon these features. They are still an important part of the RCT design. But we DO need to know this, so we don't become overly confident in a non-inferiority conclusion until we've checked a few more things.

Ask the group how we might assess the features of a non-inferiority design to make sure we feel comfortable with the level of bias. They may suggest abandoning some of the traditional RCT features. While we can't abandon randomization, equal treatment, or complete follow-up, some authors advocate repeating the analysis without intention to treat. Doing a "per-protocol" analysis after the intention-to-treat analysis may uncover differences that weren't initially evident, and may challenge the conclusion of non-inferiority. To summarize some things you can do to protect a non-inferiority trial from bias:

Plan the *POWER* calculation clearly.

Account for *DROP-OUTS* stringently, because reducing the number of events you can analyze may make non-inferiority easier to find.

Use more than one *outcome assessor*. This point is not immediately intuitive! Ask learners to imagine that there is only one outcome assessor. If that person's bias is that Drug A is truly better than Drug B for reducing events, and they are TRULY BLINDED to which group is which, can they exert their bias on the data? They really can't. Now, imagine this one outcome assessor truly believes there is no difference between the groups. Can they exert this bias? They CAN, in fact!! They could (consciously or unconsciously) "under-call" the outcome events for all participants, lowering the event rate, and reducing power. This is why it's a good idea to have more than one outcome assessor and show their level of agreement.

Add a "*per-protocol*" analysis to your intention to treat analysis. This is the most controversial of all, since adding the per-protocol analysis breaks intention-to-treat analysis and allows for bias and confounding. However, here it also serves as a sanity check on the findings. If non-inferiority is found with the intention-to-treat analysis, but A DIFFERENCE is found with the per-protocol analysis, it would call the findings into question and more data would be needed before concluding non-inferiority definitively.

Appendix

Worksheet 5.0—Critical appraisal of a non-inferiority study

Non-inferiority trial critical appraisal worksheet

Statistics	
Noninferiority Margin – clinically meaningful? based on prior studies? using most conservative historical benefit over placebo?	
Power – was it adequate and maintained? Defined a priori?	
Was superiority tested?	
Was the effect of the standard treatment preserved?	
Was the standard treatment administered optimally, in a population with adequate chance of outcomes?	
Were event rates comparable to historical trials?	
Validity – Watch out for regression to the null	
Randomized	
Allocation Concealed	
Similar at baseline	
Blinding [>1 outcome assessor?]	
Equal Treatment	
Intention to treat [Per protocol analysis added?]	
Follow-up [drop outs stringently accounted for?]	
Stopped early?	
Can i apply the results to patient care?	
Patients similar to mine? Important outcomes assessed? Benefits outweigh harms?	

References

1. US Department of Health and Human Services, Food and Drug Administration. Non-inferiority clinical trials to establish effectiveness: guidance for industry. Silver Spring: US Department of Health and Human Services, Food and Drug Administration; 2016.
2. Mulla SM, Scott IA, et al. How to use a noninferiority trial. In: Guyatt G, Rennie D, Meade MO, Cook DJ, editors. User's guides to the medical literature: a manual for evidence based clinical practice. 3rd ed. Chicago, IL: American Medical Association; 2015.
3. Mulla SM, Scott IA, et al. How to use a noninferiority trial. JAMA. 2012;308(24):2605–11.
4. D'Agostino RB Sr, Massaro JM, Sullivan LM. Non-inferiority trials: design concepts and issues—the encounters of academic consultants in statistics. Stat Med. 2003;22:169–86.
5. Piaggio G, Elbourne DR, et al., for the CONSORT Group. Reporting of noninferiority and equivalence randomized trials: an extension of the CONSORT statement. JAMA. 2006;295:1152–60.
6. Kirshner B. Methodological standards for assessing therapeutic equivalence. J Clin Epidemiol. 1991;44(8):839–49.
7. Granger CB, Alexander JH, et al. Apixaban vs Warfarin in patients with atrial fibrillation. N Engl J Med. 2011;365(11):981–92.

Harm and Causation: Assessing the Value of Studies of Harm

6

Daniella A. Zipkin and Jeffrey Kushinka

Guide for the Teacher

Harm and causation questions make up a significant portion of the medical literature, in the form of cohort and case-control studies. Teaching harm can work well in the beginning of an evidence-based medicine course, particularly during discussions of study design. The topic flows well from a review of the strengths and weaknesses of cohort and case-control studies. Harm and causation questions come up frequently in various clinical settings. In addition, because results of studies that show negative associations tend to be highlighted often by news outlets and social media, patient exposure to the results generated by these types of studies tends to be high. We recommend covering the following components when teaching harm and causation:

1. Framing a harm or causation question.
2. Selecting the optimal study design. Study selection is covered separately in Chap. 3.
3. Assessing the risk of bias in cohort and case-control studies.
4. Calculating relative risk (when possible) and odds ratios for studies of harm and causation.
5. Describing the appropriate use of odds ratios and their limitations.

D. A. Zipkin (✉)
Department of Medicine, Duke University Health System, Duke University School of Medicine, Durham, NC, USA
e-mail: daniella.zipkin@duke.edu

J. Kushinka
Department of Internal Medicine, Virginia Commonwealth University School of Medicine, Richmond, VA, USA
e-mail: Jeffrey.kushinka@vcuhealth.org

D. A. Zipkin (ed.), *Teaching Evidence-Based Medicine*,
https://doi.org/10.1007/978-3-031-11174-7_6

6. App ying the results of harm trials to individual patients.
7. Communicating the results of harm trials to patients.

For each of these sub-topics you will find:

- Core content handout—we recommend learners read ahead of class.
- Samples of articles and accompanying worksheets for exercises to do together during teaching.
- Supplementary material in some cases.
- Links to videos with examples of real time teaching.

While framing the question and selecting the design can be taught in a brief introduction (under 15 min), each of the other topics may require an hour—risk of bias, odds ratios vs. relative risk (risk ratios), applying results, and communicating results.

Study Design for Harm or Causation Questions

Determining harm or causation requires investigating associations between exposures and outcomes. Different types of studies can provide information regarding these associations. *Randomized controlled trials* are the best studies for evidence of causation, because unmeasured variables which may impact the associations will be randomly distributed throughout the subjects. However, it is not often that a randomized trial will detect unexpected harm, and naturally it is unethical to plan an RCT when harm is expected (unless you plan to *reduce* a known harm). In addition, randomized controlled trials may not be designed with a follow up period which is long enough to detect the emergence of relevant harms.

The next best study design would be a *cohort study*, where a group with the exposure or treatment is compared to a group without the exposure, and followed prospectively. However, this study design is weaker, because we are unable to control for factors that influenced who received the exposure [1]. These factors, known as *confounders,* may be driving the apparent associations, with the exposure being investigated actually having little or no impact on the outcome in question. (see a full discussion of confounding on the following page). The manner in which exposed and unexposed subjects are selected is a big determinant of confounding. *Selection bias* results when the study sample does not represent the target population because of the site of recruitment or differences in baseline demographic factors [2]. Cohort studies may suffer from *detection bias*, or the tendency to look more closely for an outcome in one group over another, based on exposure (i.e., if we look more frequently in the exposure group and therefore find an association more frequently, how do we know we are not missing the same association in the control group?). Cohort studies may also be subject to *outcome ascertainment bias*, or the tendency to identify an outcome differently in each group being compared. This can occur if we define the outcome differently in the groups, or if we look for the outcome differently in the groups.

Case-control studies begin with gathering two groups of patients based on outcome status—one group with the outcome of interest, and one without—and then looking retrospectively to determine the degree of the exposure in each group. Because the selection of patients who have had the outcome (cases) and who have not had the outcome (controls) can impact all subsequent investigation about determining the potential exposure, case-control studies are prone to a number of biases. Among these are *selection bias*, *recall bias*, and *interviewer bias*, as all case-control studies require looking back in time to assess the degree of exposure. Because of the high risk of bias in case-control studies, they should be reserved for situations where the outcome is *rare*, making a prospective cohort or randomized trial not feasible. Case-control studies should be considered "hypothesis generating," and should lead to more rigorously designed studies to confirm the findings whenever possible.

Finally, the weakest form of evidence about causation is the *case series*. This is simply a series of cases where it was noted that an exposure and an outcome had occurred, and there is no comparison group. Case series are similar to case-control studies in that they are only useful in generating hypotheses that may lead to more rigorous studies.

Confounding Variables

Confounding can be caused by any factor that is associated with both the exposure and the outcome of interest, as depicted in Fig. 6.1. Confounders may be "silently" influencing the outcome more than the exposure being studied. In order to address confounding, one must be able to:

1. Think of all potential confounders,
2. Measure the confounders to the greatest degree of accuracy possible,
3. Input a numeric value for each confounder in a complex equation known as regression analysis (while performing regression analyses is beyond the scope of

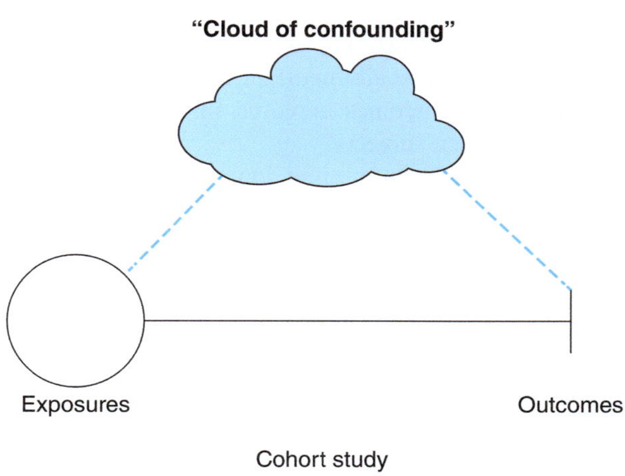

Fig. 6.1 Cohort with cloud of confounding. Confounding can be represented by a "cloud" that hovers over ever cohort. Confounders are variables which correlate with both the exposure and outcome and may be silently driving the observed association

this text, we will review important features of regression analyses to watch for as you interpret studies).

4. Assess whether the relationship between exposure and outcome persists even after adjusting for each confounder, one at a time, in the regression analysis.

Imagine a ridiculous situation with an exposure we know to be harmful: cigarette smoking. Imagine investigators wanted to assess whether cigarette smoking was a contributor to cirrhosis. Imagine these investigators found an association between cigarette smoking and cirrhosis but failed to account for the amount of alcohol consumption in these patients. We would be missing a major variable that is likely to be driving the outcome in question and lead to a potentially spurious association between cigarette smoking and cirrhosis.

Many confounders in psychosocial domains are important drivers of associations and cannot be reliably measured. Behavioral confounders, such as dietary habits, exercise, optimism, self-care, and utilization of support services are good examples of this. As a result, even studies which adjust for multiple confounding variables can never eliminate all confounding. The only way to eliminate the impact of confounding is to conduct a randomized trial, where randomization evenly distributes all confounders across the groups, including the confounders we cannot think of or cannot measure.

Assessing Bias in Studies of Harm or Causation

We take all of the factors above into account when assessing the extent of bias in a study of harm or causation (Box 6.1).

Box 6.1 Assessing the Risk of Bias in a Cohort Study

- Assessing the risk of bias in a cohort study:
  - Was the study population representative of the target population?
  - Were patients similar with respect to risk factors for the outcome, aside from the exposure of interest?
  - Was statistical adjustment for confounding variables described clearly and include all important variables?
  - Were outcomes explored in a similar fashion in exposed and non-exposed subjects?
  - Was follow-up time long enough for important outcomes to have emerged?
- Assessing the risk of bias in a case-control study.
  - Were cases and controls gathered from the same population?
  - Were cases and controls matched with regard to socio-demographic variables and clinical variables known to impact the likelihood of exposure?
  - Was the detection of exposures reliable and carried out in the same way in both groups?

TEACH IT!!

Bias in Studies of Harm or Causation

15 min:

Discussion of bias in harm studies centers around confounding. Start with a diagram on the board of a schematic of a cohort study, a circle on the left, with a horizontal line extending forward in time to the right, moving from exposures to outcomes. Above the cohort, consider drawing a "cloud" to represent confounding. The cloud should connect to both the exposures side and the outcomes side via dotted lines (Fig. 6.1).

Give the group a simple example to examine: for instance, there are cohort studies which have found associations between diet soda consumption and diabetes [3]. This isn't immediately intuitive, given the lack of sugar in diet soda, and it's not clear if there is a compound in diet soda causing the association. This example is on an accessible and familiar topic, allows the group to think about confounding, and lends itself well to a review of different sorts of confounders. Have the group brainstorm confounders in this situation—invariably, some version of the following will emerge: pre-existing obesity, socioeconomic status, diet/fast food intake, social groupings, personality factors not otherwise specified, etc.

With some confounders listed in your "cloud", remind the group that in order to adjust for confounding we must think of the confounders, measure them, and plug them into a mathematical formula called regression analysis. How easily can we measure obesity? Quite easily, use the body mass index! How easily can we measure dietary intake? This turns out to be much harder. Estimates about dietary intake are notoriously fraught with inaccuracies due to self reporting and the social expectations about dietary intake. How about social groupings? Even tougher—we can't measure that well at all.

Conclude with the point that we can NEVER eliminate confounding altogether. Studies do their best in identifying the most important confounders and adjusting for them, but it's not a perfect process. One should assume every cohort has residual confounding.

Explore other sources of bias through discussion:

What exposures would lead to more interactions with the health care system, for instance, and therefore a greater likelihood that the outcome of interest will be discovered? This is an example of detection bias.

Did outcomes have enough time to develop? If time was insufficient, and fewer outcomes are found, this will lead to imprecise estimates due to greater random error with smaller numbers.

30 min:

Add examples to the above discussion, and pre-select one or two studies for which the group can do a full assessment of bias.

If time is short, one option is to "pre-digest" the paper, highlighting key paragraphs where the answers on bias can be found. If you have more time, allow learners to read the article on the spot and then discuss.

Touch on the following concepts, through discussion as a group, and have learners take turns speaking:

Who were the patients? Do they represent a group in which this questions is important?

Were confounders fully assessed and adjusted for?

Was the outcome equally likely to be detected in those with and without the exposure?

Was follow-up complete, and was the time frame sufficient to see important outcomes?

You can use Worksheet 6.0, in the Appendix, as a guide for critical appraisal for learners.

For additional techniques on teaching adjustment for confounding, we recommend the Teaching Tips article entitled "Tips for Teachers of Evidence-Based Medicine: Adjusting for Prognostic Imbalances (Confounding Variables) in Studies on Therapy or Harm" [4].

Harm Math and the Magnitude of Association

In this section, we assess the strength of the association between exposure and outcome, ask whether or not a dose-response relationship exists, and look at the precision of the estimate. A dose-response relationship means that the magnitude of the association increases with increasing "dose," or amount, of the exposure. Precision refers to the confidence interval around the point estimate—the larger the confidence interval, the greater the variability and uncertainty of the estimate, and the lower the precision.

Definitions

$$\textbf{Odds} = \frac{(N \text{ with event})}{(N \text{ without event})}$$

$$\textbf{Risk} = \frac{(N \text{ with event})}{(\text{total } N)}$$

Table 6.1 The 2 × 2 table

	Outcome present	Outcome absent
Exposed	a	b
Not exposed	c	d

Results will usually be presented as a relative risk (RR, same as "risk ratio"), hazard ratio (HR, a more sophisticated risk ratio which accounts for changes in event accrual in the studies over time), or odds ratio (OR). We will tackle hazard ratios a little later. For now, it is important to review the differences between odds and risk, because odds ratios are always at least a little bit inflated compared to risk ratios. We intuitively think in terms of risk, so this inflation could prove deceptive when we interpret study results.

The RR is the risk in the exposed group divided by the risk in the unexposed group. The OR is the odds in the exposed group divided by the odds in the unexposed group. These are both ratios, so a value greater than 1 represents an increase in risk or odds, less than 1 a decrease in risk or odds. Remember the basic definitions of risk and odds as we move forward, beginning with Table 6.1.

Calculations

RR = [a/(a + b)]/[c/(c + d)]

OR for cohort studies (prospective: odds of outcome given certain exposure) = [a/b]/[c/d] or ad/cb

OR for case-control studies (retrospective: odds of exposure given certain outcome) = [a/c]/[b/d] or ad/cb

[Notice that mathematically, these OR calculations start in different places, but come out to be the same!]

Odds Are Always Larger Than Risk!

Odds ratios will most closely approximate risk ratios when:

- The event or outcome is rare
- The risk difference is small
- The study is large.

Compromising on these factors will cause the odds ratio to start deviating from the risk ratio, often by an unacceptably large gap.

Odds ratios are also appropriate for:

Case-control studies—When outcomes and exposures are dichotomous (i.e., they are either present or absent), they lend themselves well to calculation of odds ratios. In addition, with case-control studies, the concept of "total N," the denominator in a risk ratio, is not applicable, because we recruited an arbitrary number of study participants to make up that population.

Regression analyses—the statistical process of evaluating predictors of an outcome works best with odds ratios, because odds ratios can be multiplied and inserted into complex mathematical formulas easily. The output of a regression analysis will be an odds ratio, but authors can then choose to convert it to a risk ratio for publication. While the details of conducting regression analysis are beyond the scope of this text, knowing that the process occurs with odds ratios helps to explain why some prospective cohorts will present odds ratios for their main outcomes. One must ask why they did not convert back to risk ratios—is it possible that the inflated number suited their aims more?

How do we interpret an odds ratio or risk ratio once it is calculated? Think of it as a relative increase or decrease in odds. The math here is similar to what we reviewed in the Therapy chapter. Keep in mind that any ratio (risk ratio or odds ratio) of 1 means there is no difference between the groups being compared. Therefore, for any ratio not equal to 1, the distance from 1 tells us the relative odds or relative risk. For instance, if the odds ratio is 1.3, that represents a 30% relative increase in odds. We can't make sense of this number without knowing the baseline risk for the condition. Imagine the baseline risk is 2%. A 30% increase in that risk would move the risk from 2% to 2.6%. Thus, it is important to bring the relative change back to absolute terms. Please see Chap. 4 for an explanation of these concepts. The *number needed to harm* can be calculated in the same way as the number needed to treat—is it simply the reciprocal of the absolute risk increase. It should be noted that we cannot calculate a number needed to harm for case-control studies because they are retrospective and reflect an arbitrary number of subjects.

The *precision* of these estimates can be assessed by examining the confidence interval around the estimate. In a study which demonstrates an association between an exposure and an adverse outcome, the lower limit of the CI provides a minimal estimate of the strength of the association. In a study which has failed to demonstrate an association, the upper boundary of the CI tells you how big an adverse effect may still be present, despite the failure to show a statistically significant association.

Factors that influence *clinical decision-making* regarding harm include the strength of the association, the magnitude of the risk, the available alternatives, and the possible adverse consequences of minimizing exposure. If there is significant bias in the study design and the association is weak (OR of less than 2.0), then it is probably best to wait for other data to confirm and strengthen the finding. Nonetheless, once even a small possibility of harm exists, the ethical, legal, and societal impact may trump the evidence. Health systems may need to act on the potential harm even if "truth" has not been confirmed.

TEACH IT!!

Harm Math and Applying Results to Patients

15–20 min:

Have learners fill out the Worksheet 6.1, available in the Appendix. This compares odds and risk for different shaded portions of the pie chart. Discuss with them, and be sure they notice that as the proportion of the shaded area gets larger, odds and risk diverge more and more. The answer key is provided in Worksheet 6.2.

Move on to Worksheet 6.3 attached at the end of this chapter, or provide a similar example utilizing simple numbers. A humorous scenario never hurts! As learners move through the calculations, make the following observations as a group. We provide answers to this imaginary scenario in Worksheet 6.4 for reference.

Odds ratios, like Odds, differ from Risk Ratios when event rates are large.

Odds ratios are more inflated compared to Risk Ratios when the risk difference is larger.

For case-control studies, you cannot calculate risk ratios.

The mathematical result for a cohort study vs. a case-control study for the same dataset will be numerically the same. What differs is how you say it. Have learners practice putting the odds ratio into a sentence for both a cohort study and a case-control study. For instance, say the odds ratio is 2.5. In a cohort study, you might say "the exposed group had 2.5 times greater odds of having the outcome than the non-exposed group". In a case-control study, you might say "those with the outcome had a 2.5 times greater odds of having been exposed than those without the outcome".

10–15 min:

Follow the exercise above by looking at real world examples and interpreting the magnitude of the results. For this portion, it is ok to utilize abstracts only, rather than the full studies, because you'd like the group to look at the results and imagine how to communicate them to patients. For this exercise, you can assume the risk of bias in the selected papers was low and move straight to results.

Discuss the odds ratio or hazard ratio presented in the abstract and put it into words. This is a relative number—i.e., a "relative increase in odds" or a "relative increase in risk."

Provide a patient case around the study of interest, and estimate that patient's baseline risk for the condition. Utilize medical databases, or clinical judgment, with the scenario you have set up.

Remember that odds ratios and hazard ratios are relative increases or decreases in risk. This means that in order to assess the real magnitude, you need to determine the baseline odds or risk of the outcome, and then multiply by the relative change reflected in the ratio.

Example: a 42-year-old man with no medical history aside from persistent gastro-esophageal reflux has been stable on a proton-pump inhibitor (PPI) for several years. He recently learned that the PPI was associated with kidney failure based on a news report of a new study [5] *and stopped taking it. His acid reflux symptoms are severe again. How can you counsel him?*

> *A quick read of the abstract tells you that this well-done cohort study found an association between PPI use and incident chronic kidney disease in adults aged 63 on average. Adjusted analyses found a HR of 1.50* [5]. *How do you apply this to your patient?*

Discuss what you've learned: if we trust this study, what is the magnitude of the impact for our patient? Many studies of harm report small to moderate odds ratios. Relative increases to harms with low baseline risks will result in very small changes. These changes may or may not impact how we counsel patients about these harms! This is particularly true when all cohort studies and case-control studies struggle with bias, and these results may be subject to error. This may be an appropriate place to remind the learners about several key points: the discussion of harms in the lay media is often rather alarmist and overstates the impact of relatively small odds ratios and risk ratios, and these studies identify associations only and are NOT proof of cause and effect.

Appendix

Worksheet 6.0—Critical appraisal for studies of harm or causation

Harm and causationcriticalappraisal worksheet (cohort and case control)

Assessing the risk of bias in a cohort study	
Was the study population representative of the target population?	
Were patients similar with respect to risk factors for the outcome, aside from the exposure of interest?	
Was statistical adjustment for confounding variables described clearly with all important variables included?	
Were outcomes explored in a similar fashion in exposed and non-exposed subjects?	
Was follow-up time long enough for important outcomes to have emerged?	
Assessing the risk of bias in a case control study	
Were cases and controls gathered from the same population?	
Were cases and controls matched with regard to socio-demographic variables and clinical variables known to impact the likelihood of exposure?	
Was the detection of exposures reliable and carried out the same way in both groups?	
Assessing the results in a cohort or case control study	
What is the magnitude and precision of the results?	
Can the results be applied to my patient population?	

Worksheet 6.1—Odds exercise, blank

Risk vs. Odds comparison

$$\text{Risk} = \frac{\text{N\_event}}{\text{Total N}}$$

$$\text{Odds} = \frac{\text{N\_event}}{\text{N\_without\_event}}$$

As the frequency of an event increases, what do you notice about the risk and the odds of that event?

	Risk	Odds
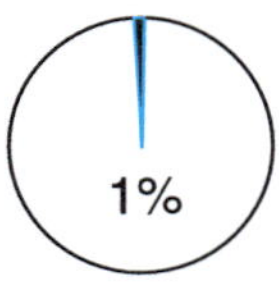		
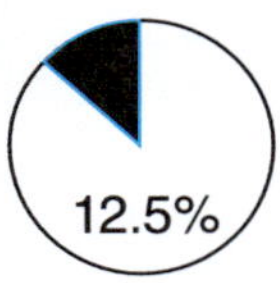		
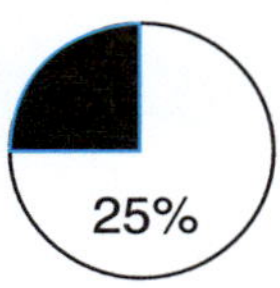		
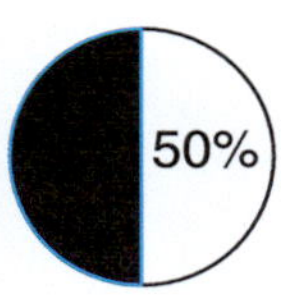		
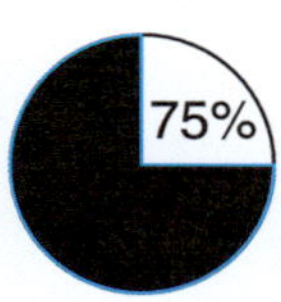		

Worksheet 6.2—Odds exercise, answers

Risk vs. Odds comparison- Answers

Risk = $\frac{\text{N\_event}}{\text{Total N}}$

Odds = $\frac{\text{N\_event}}{\text{N\_without\_event}}$

As the frequency of an event increases, odds and risk diverge more and more, with odds becoming unacceptably inflated. We should only rely on odds for rare events.

	Risk	Odds
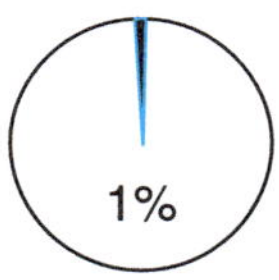	$\frac{1}{100} = 0.01$	1:99 = 0.010101…
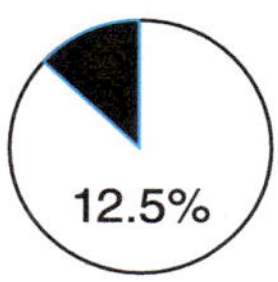	$\frac{12.5}{100} = 0.125$	12.5:87.5 = 0.143
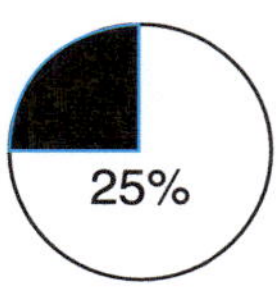	$\frac{25}{100} = 0.25$	25:75 = 0.33
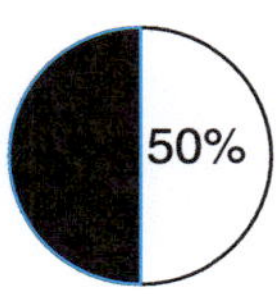	$\frac{50}{100} = 0.5$	50:50 = 1
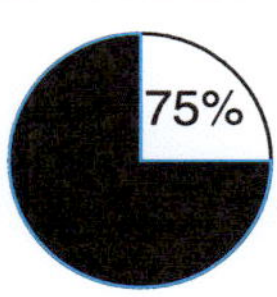	$\frac{75}{100} = 0.75$	75:25 = 3

Worksheet 6.3—Odds ratio exercise, blank

Odds Ratios can be inflated too!

The Case: You are at a large family picnic when your second cousin once removed, Jack, comes up to you and asks your help settling a medical question. He thinks that the best way to avoid a major belly ache after the picnic is to eat only hot dogs, which are a new offering this year, but your great aunt Millie thinks it's best to eat only hamburgers like they did in the old days. Because you are an ambitious student of EBM, you immediately design a study. You enroll everyone at the picnic who chose either hot dogs or hamburgers, and you arrange to call everyone the next morning to gather data…

	Outcome: Belly Ache	No Outcome: Feeling great!
Exposure: Hot Dogs	40	60
Control: Hamburgers	20	80

Relative Risk (RR) of Hot Dog consumption leading to belly ache:

RR = Risk with Hot Dog/Risk with Hamburger =

Odds Ratio (OR) of Hot Dog consumption leading to belly ache:

OR = Odds with Hot Dog/Odds with Hamburger =

What do you notice?

You decide to look at this important question again at next year's picnic, because your EBM teacher said all studies should be replicated! Here is the data gathered this time:

	Outcome: Belly Ache	No Outcome: Feeling great!
Exposure: Hot Dog	30	70
Control: Hamburger	25	75

Relative Risk (RR):

RR =

Odds ratio (OR):

OR =

What do you notice, now? What happened as we narrowed the risk difference?

In year three, you get a bit of a late start planning, so you decide to perform this research in a different way. You get the full family phone list the day after the picnic, and then call each person to ask them if they have a belly ache, and what they ate.

What is the name of this study design? ____________________

Shockingly, your numbers come out looking very similar to the last set. Recalculate the Odds Ratio only, now from the vantage point of this new study design, moving backwards from outcomes to exposures. **(Why are we only calculating the Odds Ratio, and not a Risk Ratio this time?)**

	Outcome: Belly Ache	No Outcome: Feeling great!
Exposure: Hot Dogs	30	70
Control: Hamburgers	25	75

Odds ratio (OR):

OR = Odds in belly ache group/Odds in feeling great group =

What do you notice?

Try to speak the results of this study in a sentence! Compare that to how you would speak the results of the previous study.

Worksheet 6.4—Odds ratio exercise, answers

Odds Ratios can be inflated too!

The Case: You are at a large family picnic when your second cousin once removed, Jack, comes up to you and asks your help settling a medical question. He thinks that the best way to avoid a major belly ache after the picnic is to eat only hot dogs, which are a new offering this year, but your great aunt Millie thinks it's best to eat only hamburgers like they did in the old days. Because you are an ambitious student of EBM, you immediately design a study. You enroll everyone at the picnic who chose either hot dogs or hamburgers, and you arrange to call everyone the next morning to gather data…

	Outcome: Belly Ache	No Outcome: Feeling great!
Exposure: Hot Dogs	40	60
Control: Hamburgers	20	80

Relative Risk (RR) of Hot Dog consumption leading to belly ache:

RR = Risk with Hot Dog/Risk with Hamburger = (40/100)/(20/100) = 2.0

Odds Ratio (OR) of Hot Dog consumption leading to belly ache:

OR = Odds with Hot Dog/Odds with Hamburger = (40/60)/(20/80) = 2.67

What do you notice? The estimate is inflated when using odds! Why? Because it's not a rare event, and it's not a large population.

You decide to look at this important question again at next year's picnic, because your EBM teacher said all studies should be replicated! Here is the data gathered this time:

	Outcome: Belly Ache	No Outcome: Feeling great!
Exposure: Hot Dog	30	70
Control: Hamburger	25	75

Relative Risk (RR):

RR = (30/100)/(25/100) = 1.2

Odds ratio (OR):

OR = (30/70)/(25/75) = 1.29

What do you notice, now? What happened as we narrowed the risk difference? Still inflated, but less so. Why? Even with a relatively common event, risk difference will also play into how inflated the odds ratio can get.

In year three, you get a bit of a late start planning, so you decide to perform this research in a different way. You get the full family phone list the day after the picnic, and then call each person to ask them if they have a belly ache, and what they ate.

What is the name of this study design? Case-control!

Shockingly, your numbers come out looking very similar to the last set. Recalculate the Odds Ratio only, now from the vantage point of this new study design, moving backwards from outcomes to exposures. **(Why are we only calculating the Odds Ratio, and not a Risk Ratio this time?** Because we cannot calculate Risk in a case control – there is no "total N" for the denominator, we selected the population ourselves…**)**

	Outcome: Belly Ache	No Outcome: Feeling great!
Exposure: Hot Dogs	30	70
Control: Hamburgers	25	75

Odds ratio (OR):

OR = Odds in belly ache group/Odds in feeling great group =
(30/25)/(70/75) = 1.29

What do you notice? 1.29 is exactly the same as the last time was calculated this!

It turns out, the math doesn't change if you are a cohort study or a retrospective case control study. It is the same either way – all that changes is how you communicate those results.

Try to speak the results of this study in a sentence! Compare that to how you would speak the results of the previous study.

In the case control version, we say "those with belly ache had a 1.29 greater odds of having eaten hot dogs".

In the cohort version on the previous page, we say "those who ate hot dogs had a 1.29 greater odds of having a belly ache".

References

1. Grimes DA, Shulz KF. Bias and causal associations in observational research. Lancet. 2002;359:248–52.
2. Ellenberg JH. Cohort studies: selection bias in observational and experimental studies. Stat Med. 1994;13:557–67.
3. Nettleton JA, Lutsey PL, et al. Diet soda intake and risk of incident metabolic syndrome and type 2 diabetes in the Multi-Ethnic Study of Atherosclerosis (MESA). Diabetes Care. 2009;32(4):688–94.
4. Kennedy CC, Jaeschke R, et al. Tips for teachers of evidence-based medicine: adjusting for prognostic imbalances (confounding variables) in studies on therapy or harm. J Gen Intern Med. 2008;23(3):337–43.
5. Lazarus B, Chen Y, et al. Proton pump inhibitor use and the risk of chronic kidney disease. JAMA Intern Med. 2016;176(2):238–46.

Diagnostic Testing: Assessing the Value of Studies of Diagnostic Tests

7

Daniella A. Zipkin and Kathleen W. Bartlett

Guide for the Teacher

This section covers the interpretation of studies of diagnostic tests. These studies are typically cross-sectional, where the test in question is applied to all patients, and a gold standard is applied to all patients, and the two are compared. Most learners tend to be familiar with the ideas of sensitivity and specificity, as these constructs are classically taught and included on standardized tests. We recommend not only shifting the conversation to likelihood ratios as the most reliable single metric of a test result's value, but also framing it in terms of how the test result alters pre-test probability. Learners should assess pre-test probability before they begin, decide that testing is appropriate, apply the likelihood ratio to their pre-test probability to determine a post-test probability, and then assess how the test result ultimately affected their clinical decision making. We recommend covering the following components when teaching diagnosis:

Supplementary Information The online version contains supplementary material available at [https://doi.org/10.1007/978-3-031-11174-7_7].

D. A. Zipkin (✉)
Department of Medicine, Duke University Health System,
Duke University School of Medicine, Durham, NC, USA
e-mail: daniella.zipkin@duke.edu

K. W. Bartlett
Department of Pediatrics, Duke Children's Hospital, Duke University, Durham, NC, USA
e-mail: katy.bartlett@duke.edu

D. A. Zipkin (ed.), *Teaching Evidence-Based Medicine*,
https://doi.org/10.1007/978-3-031-11174-7_7

1. Framing a diagnosis question.
2. Assessing the risk of bias of diagnostic testing studies, particularly spectrum bias.
3. Calculating sensitivity, specificity, and likelihood ratios for diagnostic tests. Demonstrating that likelihood ratios can be calculated for different levels of the test.
4. Applying likelihood ratios to pre-test probability to demonstrate the transition to post-test probability of disease.
5. Applying results of diagnosis trials to clinical decision making.
6. Communicating results of diagnosis studies to patients.

For each of these sub-topics you will find:

- Core content handout—we recommend learners read ahead of class.
- Samples of articles and accompanying worksheets for exercises to do together during teaching.
- Supplementary material in some cases.
- Links to videos with examples of real time teaching.

Framing the question and selecting the design can be taught in a brief introduction (under 15 min). Assessing for bias, in particular spectrum bias, can be taught in a 30 min small group session. Calculating likelihood ratios and applying them to pre-test probability can be taught in 60–90 min.

Diagnostic Testing Study Design and Sources of Bias

A diagnostic test can be any aspect of the clinical encounter that is used to differentiate between possible diagnoses—it can be an element of the history or physical, a blood or urine test, an imaging study, etc. Studies about diagnostic tests are generally *cross-sectional or cohort* studies, where all subjects receive both the test in question and the reference standard test, and the results are compared. Several core principles in the design of these studies are critical in generating results which are accurate and precise.

What is meant by the *reference standard*, also known as *gold standard* test, to which we will compare our test? The gold standard should be the best possible mechanism currently available to assess the presence or absence of disease. Gold standards are often invasive, time consuming, or expensive. Interestingly, a gold standard can itself never be verified against any other test, since it is viewed as the best test. We must be careful to ensure that the gold standard is clinically the best and most thorough test.

The next thing to consider in diagnostic testing is the patient population. The population must have a broad enough *spectrum* of disease for us to be able to ask the question of whether disease is present, considering the pathologic, clinical, and co-morbid features of the disease [1]. If the disease state is obvious and dichotomous, such that you could make the diagnosis without a test, employing a test in that population will yield no useful information. Say, for instance, you are interested in a test for dementia and you implement it in a memory care unit at a skilled nursing facility. There is no diagnostic uncertainty there, as there is a very high rate of dementia. You are asking your test to perform in an environment which is "too easy." You are not putting the test to the test! In other words, you should begin with a population in whom the diagnostic dilemma exists. In the case of the dementia scale, that may mean a population of patients over 60 with a memory concern.

The next critical element of diagnostic testing studies involves ensuring that the test and the gold standard are completely *independent* [1]. Imagine what might occur if our test were also a part of the gold standard. We would overestimate the performance of our test. Imagine what would occur if our test results influenced whether or not a patient received the gold standard test. In this case, we are already acting clinically based on the result of the first test, rather than accurately testing its performance against the gold standard. In these scenarios, estimates of test accuracy will be inaccurate, and imprecise. Blinding of the person interpreting the test to the gold standard results and vice versa is also part of keeping them independent: people tend to adjust their perceptions based on the additional data. The sources of bias discussed above are summarized in (Box 7.1).

Box 7.1 Common Biases in Diagnostic Testing

Spectrum Bias

Failure to include a properly broad, representative sample of a population with diagnostic uncertainty in a study of a diagnostic test can result in misleading estimates of sensitivity and specificity and limit applicability. We must strive for breadth with regard to pathology (extent, location, cell type), clinical features (chronicity, severity), and comorbidities. Choosing patients with unequivocally advanced disease and those who are absolutely disease-free will lead to making it easier for the test to differentiate disease or no disease. Sensitivity and specificity will look great, but may fail in a population with uncertainty!

Verification Bias

Also called "workup bias," this is any deviation in the tendency to pursue the ultimate diagnosis in patients based on other results. As patients with negative preliminary tests or low suspicion of disease are not fully worked up, sensitivity will be artificially inflated. The remedy for this type of bias is to be certain that all subjects receive gold standard assessment, regardless of other tests.

Diagnostic-Review Bias

The tendency to interpret a gold standard test with knowledge of previous testing will lead to erroneous results. Blinding is the only way to ensure that the ultimate diagnosis is made without the influence of prior test results.

Incorporation Bias
When the results of the test are incorporated into the gold standard assessment of the true diagnosis, the test cannot be separately and independently assessed for accuracy. [Food for thought: does knowledge of the clinical concern influence what the radiologist sees on a chest X-ray?]

In summary, to ensure the diagnostic testing study is free of bias, one must start with a mixed population in which there is diagnostic uncertainty. The gold standard should be the most appropriate test possible and should be independent (not related clinically or statistically) of the test itself. The gold standard must be applied to all subjects regardless of the results of the test.

TEACH IT!!

Bias in Diagnostic Testing: Spectrum Bias [2]

5–10 min

Discuss spectrum bias in the context of a clinical question or diagnostic test article. Ask the learners to assess if the spectrum is broad enough to test the test.

Draw two bell curves on the board to represent two populations of patients, one with and one without disease. Draw it once where the two curves are far apart, barely touching, then draw it again where the two curves have a lot of overlap. The *Y* axis represents number of patients, and the *X*-axis represents disease spectrum. Ask learners to discuss how a diagnostic test is likely to perform in the two scenarios. Lead them towards the idea that the further apart the two populations are, and the less overlap between them, the easier it gets for any test to tell them apart. Therefore, bi-modal populations are not a good starting point for assessing a test. There must be overlap between the populations to have diagnostic uncertainty.

Many tests are initially tested in environments that are bi-modal, as above, in the early exploratory stages. A test must, at the minimum, be able to distinguish a population with a disease from that without it, so a bi-modal population is a reasonable starting place. (If a test does NOT distinguish between two obvious groups, we can probably stop there). This is not sufficient, however, to put the test into use. It must then be tested in a mixed population where there is more overlap, and uncertainty.

15–30 min

Create a clinical scenario where developing a diagnostic test is needed. (Consider utilizing something like pulmonary sarcoidosis as an example—it has a reasonable differential diagnosis, and there is no currently available non-invasive test that correlates well with tissue biopsy.) Ask the group to build a cohort of patients in which the spectrum of disease would be sufficiently broad to "test the test". Where would patients be recruited, and how? Learners will quickly realize that every decision they make plays into the spectrum they will achieve, with patients recruited in sub-specialty environments having a narrowing spectrum. The population we use when "testing a test" will determine which populations we apply the test to. If a test is evaluated in a referral population, it may not apply to a primary care population, for instance.

30 min

Consider reviewing a full article with learners, with the critical appraisal Worksheet 7.0 as a guide, available in the Appendix.

Pretest Probability

As we approach a patient whose diagnosis we are trying to clarify, we first start with the *pretest probability*—our suspicion of how likely the disease is in this patient. Pretest probability begins with the *prevalence* of disease in patients similar to ours. We estimate prevalence by using the medical literature, clinical prediction rules, local data, and our clinical judgment. Go ahead and look at the epidemiology section of your medical reference site, for example, to get a starting point for prevalence, and then adjust based on the patient's presentation. Naturally, there can be wide variability in clinicians' estimates of pretest probability for the same patient and same condition. This tends to be a process involving both art and science!

If there are no clear references to guide you, try this exercise: Force your diagnostic options to add up to 100%. List the items on the differential, and assign them each a numeric probability, to compare and rank them. Your clinical judgment is worth a lot! *We will soon demonstrate that your pretest probability is even more important than the test you choose, when it comes to decision making.*

Test and Treatment Thresholds in the Diagnostic Process

Do we even need to perform the test in the first place? Once you know the pretest probability of a certain diagnosis, you should decide where it falls along this spectrum, as depicted in Fig. 7.1. *If the probability of disease is so low that even a positive diagnostic test would not push you to treat*—don't order the test!! *If the probability of disease is exceedingly high, such that even a negative diagnostic test will not stop you from treating*—skip the test and proceed with treatment!! In the intermediate probability areas we need the diagnostic testing to help with our management.

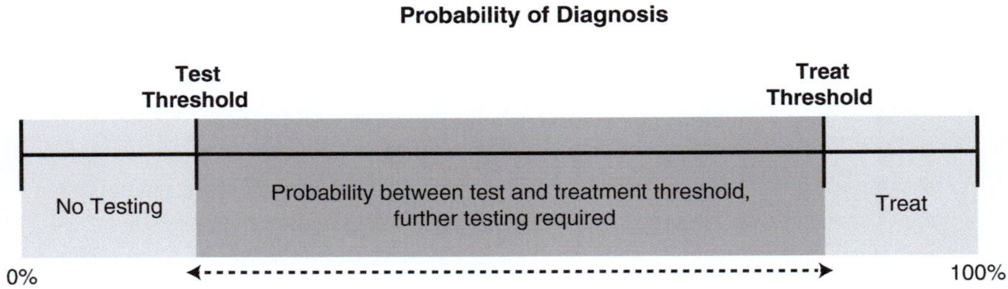

Fig. 7.1 Test and treat thresholds. Schematic demonstration of where diagnostic testing is needed—when probability of disease is above our test threshold, and below the treat threshold. The specific locations of these thresholds will vary based on the clinical condition, the consequences of missing the diagnosis, and the harms of treating or not treating

Where you place the test and treat thresholds will vary with the clinical condition, the adverse sequelae involved in missing the diagnosis, the benefits of treating and the harms associated with the treatment. The more serious a missed diagnosis, the lower the test threshold. The higher the risk associated with the diagnostic test itself, the higher the test threshold. Similarly, with the treat threshold, the greater the adverse effects of treating, the higher the threshold will be.

TEACH IT!!

Pre-test Probability

5–10 min

Ask the group what "pre-test probability" means and discuss the definition. Touch on the concept of prevalence—there is a known prevalence or probability of the condition in the population of interest, and as soon as you interact with a patient clinically you are toggling up and down in terms of that probability as you incorporate information about the history and physical exam.

Prevalence information can come from the epidemiology section of references on the condition of interest, observational or experimental studies which involve estimates of prevalence in that population, or clinical prediction rules which are widely available on apps which calculate the risk of a condition. Consider adding an exercise here of having the students search various online references for prevalence estimates from the literature.

15–30 min

Create an interactive exercise to demonstrate the variability in estimates of pre-test probability. This exercise works best in a group of at least 10 participants, the more the better. Prepare a real or fabricated case ahead of time where there is a reasonable differential diagnosis. Ask the participants to write down their estimate of probability of a specific condition, given the case at hand.

Using a dry erase board in a small group, overhead projector in a large group, or interactive space in virtual teaching formats, draw out a frequency table of the estimates of prevalence within the group, with 0–100 along one axis in increments of 10, and then dots or lines to indicate a vote. Ask each participant to share their pre-test probability. Typically, a rough bell curve will emerge, with votes converging around the most popular estimate.

Discuss that pre-test probability can be a range and can be a little subjective, but that honing your idea of pre-test probability before you launch into diagnostic testing is critical! We must know where we began in order to determine where we end up after testing.

Alternatively, create a case example which utilizes a clinical prediction rule, and have participants calculate the pre-test probability with their smart phones. Ask the group if they would adjust that estimate either up or down based on factors that are not incorporated into the rule.

Understanding the Results or Diagnostic Testing Math

Before we order a test, we are interested in the sensitivity and specificity of that test as used in previous populations that are similar to our patient. *Sensitivity* is defined as the proportion of patients with a disorder who have a positive result and *Specificity* is defined as the proportion of patients without a disorder who have a negative result. Sensitivity and specificity do not help us to determine our patient's probability of disease once we have the result. Remember, they were generated knowing the disease status via the gold standard, and we do not know our patient's disease status.

Once the diagnostic test has been ordered, you will sometimes see predictive values calculated. *Positive predictive value* is the proportion of patients with a positive test result who have the disease. *Negative predictive value* is the proportion of patients with a negative test result who don't have the disease. Positive and negative predictive values carry major limitations. The predictive value varies with the prevalence of disease in the population being studied. If you have a population with a very high prevalence of disease, the number with a positive test who have disease goes up, and the number with a positive test who don't have disease goes down—increasing the numerator of the positive predictive value and decreasing the denominator, thus inflating the positive predictive value. Keep in mind that the test itself is not changing—it is simply being applied in a new context, and suddenly the results may carry a very different meaning. It is for this reason that we prefer to focus on *likelihood ratios* [3], which are a characteristic of the test and essentially do not change as the prevalence changes.

Likelihood ratios are the most clinically useful way to represent results of diagnostic testing studies. *The likelihood ratio is the proportion of patients WITH disease with a given diagnostic test result over the proportion of patients WITHOUT disease with that test result.* The higher the likelihood ratio, the greater the increase in probability of disease given that level of the test. (See the calculations below).

A Diagnostic Dilemma

Let us use a clinical example as we go through some calculations: You are seeing a 45-year-old man for a routine physical. On questioning about alcohol use, he says that he has two to three drinks per day. He has tried to cut down in the past and feels irritable when his wife nags him about his drinking—he's answered positively to two CAGE questions. The CAGE questions are frequently used to rule in or rule out alcohol dependency. Now that he's answered two questions positively, what are the chances he is alcoholic?

You go to the literature and find an article entitled "Screening for Alcohol Abuse Using CAGE Scores and Likelihood Ratios" [4]. Sounds good! They studied 821 patients in an outpatient clinic and compared CAGE scores to the DSM-III-R (Diagnostic and Statistical Manual of Mental Disorders). Their results are represented in Table 7.1 below:

Prevalence

Prevalence = disease/total population, or (a + c)/(a + b + c + d)

$$\textit{Prevalence of alcoholism in study} = 216 + 78 / 821 = 36\%$$

Remember that prevalence is the proportion of disease in our population. It helps us determine pre-test probability, or our suspicion of disease in an individual patient before we order the test. The extent to which a test is able to adjust our probability of disease is the topic of interest. If we start with a suspicion of 36%, and a positive test moves that to 45%, it has not done much for our decision-making—we are left with more ambiguity. If it moves the probability to 90%, it is a great test and helps us a lot! The discussion of likelihood ratios below is intended to show you how a test moves that probability around.

Table 7.1 2 × 2 table for diagnostic testing math and the CAGE example for alcoholism

	Disease present	Disease absent		Alcoholic	Not alcoholic
Test positive	True pos a	False pos b	CAGE 2 or more positive	216	45
Test negative	c False neg	d True neg	CAGE 1 or less	78	482

The calculations of sensitivities and specificities are shown for historical purposes only! While you should understand the meaning of these metrics below, the likelihood ratio is the focus of using diagnostic test results:

Sensitivity and Specificity

$$\textit{Sensitivity} = \textit{in disease, the proportion with a positive test}; \mathrm{a/(a+c)}$$

$$\textit{Specificity} = \textit{without disease, proportion with a negative test}; \mathrm{d/(d+b)}$$

If 2 or more responses is cutoff:

$$\text{Sensitivity of CAGE} = 216 / 294 = 74\%$$

$$\text{Specificity of CAGE} = 482 / 527 = 91\%$$

In other words, using "2 questions answered positively" as our cutoff, someone with alcoholism has a 74% chance of having a positive CAGE test, and someone without alcoholism has a 91% chance of having a negative CAGE test. Notice that this hinges on the diagnosis after it is already known and does not tell us anything about the probability of disease in OUR patient!

Predictive Value (for *this* Population, with *this* Prevalence)

Positive predictive value (PPV) = in positive test, the proportion with disease, or a/(a + b).

If 2 or more responses is cutoff:

$$\text{PPV} = 216 / 261 = 83\%$$

Negative predictive value (NPV) = in negative test, the proportion without disease, or d/(c + d).

$$\text{NPV} = 482 / 560 = 86\%$$

In other words, for those with 2 or more questions positive, there is an 83% chance that they are alcoholic, and for those with 1 or fewer positive, there is an 86% chance that they are not alcoholic. Notice that this starts with the *test result*, not the patient!

Remember that *predictive value changes with prevalence!* In this example, the characteristics of the CAGE test don't change, but if we take this test and use it in a population with a low prevalence of alcoholism, more positives will be false positives, naturally, and the positive predictive value will go down. The test has not changed, only the population has. We will discuss another way of thinking about this below.

Back to Likelihood Ratios!!

The likelihood ratio is, for a given level of the diagnostic test, the proportion of patients WITH disease with that test result over the proportion of patients WITHOUT disease with that test result. Remember, it is always *"WITH disease over WITHOUT disease," no matter what the test result.*

In contrast to sensitivity and specificity, which are defined for dichotomous test results which are either positive or negative, likelihood ratios can be calculated for multiple levels of a test, as is illustrated in Table 7.2 regarding the CAGE questions.

When we collapse the above results into "positive" and "negative" with respect to a certain cutoff, as in the 2 × 2 table printed again below, it just so happens that the LR can be calculated from sensitivity and specificity, as given in Table 7.3:

LR of a positive test: [a/(a + c)]/[b/(b + d)]; or sens/(1-spec); or (true pos rate)/(false pos rate)

$$\text{LR of "positive" CAGE} = 0.74 / (1 - 0.91) = 8.2$$

In other words, using 2 questions or more as our cutoff, a positive CAGE test is 8.2 times more likely to occur in a person WITH alcoholism than in a person WITHOUT alcoholism.

We calculated the likelihood ratio from the sensitivity and specificity in this case because, when we dichotomized the test to either 2 or more questions positive or 0-1 positive, the likelihood of someone with alcoholism having 2 or more questions positive compared to someone without alcoholism is the same as the sensitivity over 1-specificity. However, sensitivity and specificity are NOT needed in order to calculate the LR. We will cover this in more detail in the TEACH IT section titled "Likelihood Ratios: Calculating them for different levels of a test".

Table 7.2 Likelihood ratios and multiple levels of the test, for CAGE questions

+CAGE questions	Alcoholism	No alcoholism	Likelihood ratio [calc.]
0	33	428	0.14 [(33/294)/(428/527)]
1	45	54	1.5 [(45/294)/(54/527)]
2	86	34	4.5 [(86/294)/(34/527)]
3	74	10	13 [(74/294)/(10/527)]
4	56	1	100 [(56/294)/(1/527)]
Total	294	527	

Table 7.3 Calculating LR from sensitivity and specificity

	Alcoholism	No alcoholism
CAGE 2 or more positive	216 a	45 b
CAGE 1 or less	c 78	d 482

Likelihood ratios can be calculated for negative test results as well:

LR of a *negative* test: $[c/(a + c)]/[d/(b + d)]$;
or (1-sens)/spec,
or (false neg rate)/(true neg rate).

Remember, in calculating a negative likelihood ratio, all we are doing is calculating a likelihood ratio for a different level of the test, in this case "negative." The negative likelihood ratio is *still* defined as *the proportion of patients WITH disease with that test result over the proportion of patients WITHOUT disease with that test result.* It just so happens that it is also *1-sensitivity over specificity*, when the test result is dichotomized into "positive" or "negative."

Now, let us get to the point of how we use the likelihood ratio to affect our clinical decisions. *The likelihood ratio allows us to convert from pre-test probability to post-test probability.* We can use a nomogram to go directly from pretest probability to posttest probability! The LR is a "machine" that converts what we thought the chance of disease was before, to the chance of disease now, given a certain test result.

How good does the likelihood ratio have to be? In general, a positive LR between 5 and 10 is moderate to strong, and greater than 10 is very strong, in terms of impact on shifting the probability of disease. A negative LR between 0.2 and 0.1 is moderate and below 0.1 is very strong. However, these rough guides are not at all set in stone as everything falls along a spectrum. It is easiest to look at the *nomogram* shown in Fig. 7.2, imagine scenarios with a particular pretest probability, and imagine what different LRs would do to help your uncertainty.

Using the Fagan nomogram: Find your pre-test probability on the left-hand side, the LR in the center, and connect with a straight line to the right hand side where you will find the posttest probability of disease, given that test result in that patient.

After doing this with a clinical example, ask yourself if the change between pre-test probability and post-test probability is clinically meaningful to you, and alters your management.

Try this on the nomogram: What happens if you use the CAGE questions in a population with a much lower or much higher prevalence of alcoholism? Imagine a pre-test probability for alcoholism of 10%, and then 90% (can you imagine places with very low or very high prevalence of alcoholism?). What are your post-test probabilities of disease in those situations? Did you need to do the test at all? *Now we come full circle! This is why our pre-test probability should guide our testing threshold, or help us decide whether or not we need to test in the first place. At very low pre-test probabilities, we shouldn't subject the patient to a test. At very high pre-test probabilities, we shouldn't test, we should treat.*

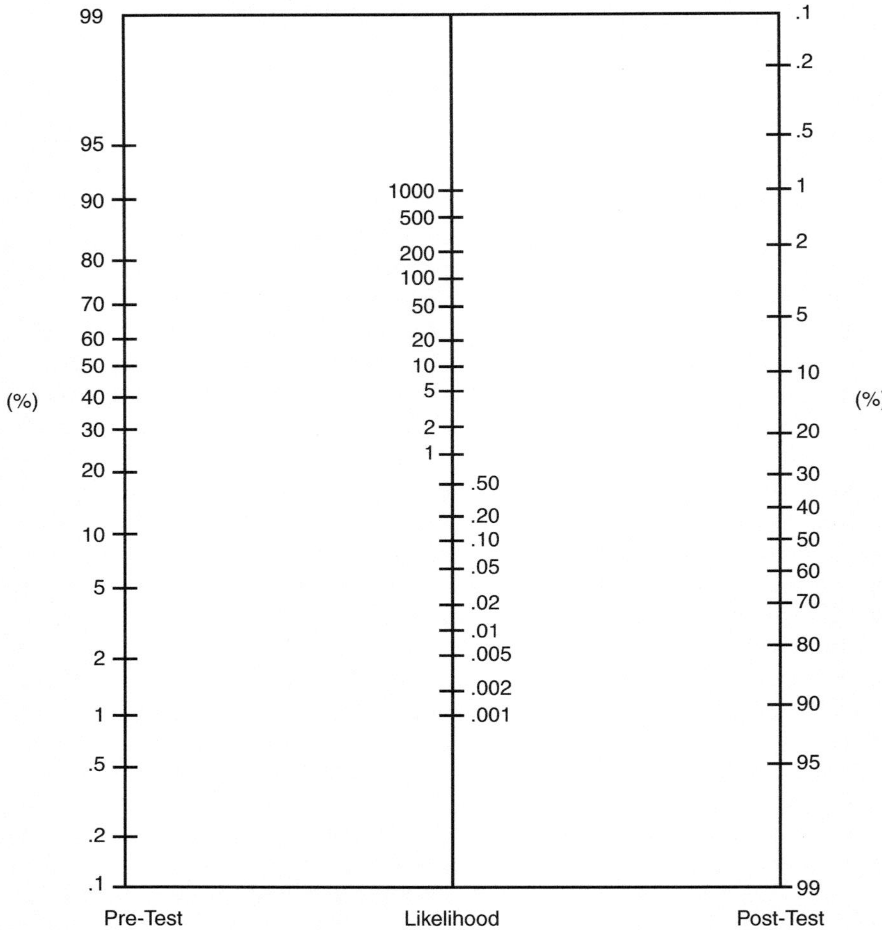

Fig. 7.2 The Fagan Nomogram [5] (used with permission from the Massachusetts Medical Society)

For the Mathematically Inclined

Here, we will review the math behind the nomogram. We cannot multiply the likelihood ratio directly by the pre-test probability, because the pre-test probability contains the numerator in both the numerator and the denominator. Instead, we need to convert pre-test probability to pre-test odds, multiply the likelihood ratio by this number, and then convert the post-test odds back to post-test probability. Here are the basic calculations:

$$[\textit{pretest probability}]/[1-\text{pretest probability}]=[\text{pretest odds}]$$
$$[\text{pretest odds}]\times[\textit{likelihood ratio}]=[\text{posttest odds}]$$
$$[\text{posttest odds}]/[\text{posttest odds}+1]=[\textit{posttest probability}]$$

For example, let us say you are treating a patient with chest pain in the ER. She is a 56-year-old woman with hypertension and a history of tobacco use, and her chest pain is dull, substernal, and present at rest for the past 2 h. You decide that the probability of her chest pain representing an MI right now is about 30% (based on published decision aids and your gut instincts.) Her EKG shows lateral 1 mm ST depression—and you learn that the likelihood ratio associated with this finding is approximately 4. Therefore, her pretest odds of MI are (0.30/0.70), or 0.43. Her posttest odds of MI are (0.43 × 4) or 1.72. Therefore, her posttest probability of MI is (1.72/2.72), or 63%. Is this probability sufficient to merit further testing and conservative treatment? Yes, indeed! So, she is admitted for observation and preventive therapy, and serum troponins are ordered, leading to further discrimination of her probability of having an MI.

Likelihood Ratios Are Generally STABLE Across Changes in Prevalence

Take a look at the 2 × 2 table again. Notice that, as prevalence increases, the proportion of patients WITH disease increases, and this will be transmitted down to both the patients WITH disease with a POSITIVE test, and the patients WITH disease with a NEGATIVE test. Similarly, those WITHOUT disease will be fewer, and this will transmit down to those WITHOUT disease with both POSITIVE and NEGATIVE tests. *If the change in prevalence affects the different levels of the test to the same degree, then the likelihood ratio will not change*. However, there is an exception to this situation. *If the spectrum of disease also changes as prevalence changes, then the LR will also change* [3]. In other words, if, along with the shift in prevalence, there is a shift towards sicker cases or other features that are picked up in different proportions by our test, then the LR cannot be used reliably across these populations. Typically, we assume that prevalence changes are not accompanied by major changes in spectrum, but we will occasionally be in error. Sometimes, the only way to know is to repeat the study in the new population. At the end of the day, *SPECTRUM of disease is the most important determinant of the resulting accuracy of the likelihood ratio.*

As a rough guide to using LRs across different prevalence populations, eyeball the populations themselves. Were they essentially the same sorts of patients, but one group had more comorbidities or a higher burden of disease? If so, it's probably safe to apply the same LR. Were they looking at patients at a different course of disease, for instance stage I-II cancers vs. stage IV? In that case, spectrum has probably shifted and LRs may not be reliable.

Use of Tests in Sequence

When more than one step in the diagnostic process is required, and multiple tests are used to establish a diagnosis, likelihood ratios are applied in sequence. The posttest probability from the first test can be used as the pretest probability for the next test, and the calculations are then repeated. This is only true, however, if the two tests in question are statistically independent—meaning that the result of one bears no relationship to the result of another. If tests are in fact dependent on each other (for instance, the results of a nuclear stress test may be dependent on the results of an EKG stress test), then data accounting for their concordance must be used to sort out the post-test probabilities. This requires data from the literature which tell us patient outcomes with both tests positive, and with one or both tests negative. While we will rarely do these calculations in real time, we are generally forming our posttest probabilities and thresholds for treatment as test results stack up, which together form a picture of the most likely diagnosis.

If the criterion for statistical independence between the two tests in sequence is met, then, mathematically, it is acceptable to multiply two likelihood ratios together and use it as one number. Try it out—pick a pre-test probability and move through one LR to get a post-test probability, then take that new probability and move through the next LR. You will end up in the same place as if you had started with the first pre-test probability and moved through the multiplied LR. For instance: pre-test probability is 30%, go through LR of 2 to get to 45%. Then take 45% and go through LR of 5 to get close to 80% post-test probability. This is the same as if we had started at 30% and gone through an LR of 10 (2 × 5), to also get to close to 80%.

TEACH IT!!

Sensitivity and Specificity

Teachers of Evidence Based Medicine take different approaches to the topic of sensitivity and specificity. Inherent features of any test with dichotomous outcomes, sensitivity and specificity made up the bulk of teaching and testing on the topic of diagnosis in the past. However, they do not help us apply a diagnostic test result to a patient to better understand that patient's probability of disease. In this teaching section, we take the approach of reviewing sensitivity and specificity for the learner up front, moving to incorporating them into the formation of likelihood ratios, and ultimately abandoning them as we teach how likelihood ratios can be calculated for multiple levels of a test, not only dichotomous ("positive" or "negative") tests. We have chosen to start with these familiar concepts because they are still prevalent in the literature, clinical discourse, and standardized testing. In addition, some more experienced learners may be able to state that the LR is "sensitivity over one minus specificity", but often can't say why.

For this session and the sessions on likelihood ratios that follow, we recommend using the paper on ferritin as a test for iron deficiency in the elderly [6], because the numbers are simple and the data provide an opportunity to learn all the facets of likelihood ratios.

5–10 min:

Draw a 2 × 2 table on the dry erase board for a small group session, or create slides with a 2 × 2 table for a large group session. *If you are using the ferritin paper above, use a ferritin below 45 for your cutoff for a "positive" test and above 45 for your cutoff for a "negative" test, for this portion of the lesson.* Use Worksheets 7.1 and 7.2, found in the Appendix, as guides for this exercise.

Ask the learners to define sensitivity and specificity. Review how both sensitivity and specificity begin WITH KNOWLEDGE OF DISEASE. We must already have confirmed who has disease and who does not, using a gold standard, in order to calculate sensitivity and specificity. This is one reason why they are not helpful when we are curious about whether our patient has a disease.

As you define sensitivity, draw an arrow moving down the left column of your 2 × 2 table, in a contrasting color, and label it "sensitivity". This arrow represents the formula: all those with disease who have a positive test, over all those with disease. See an example in Fig. 7.3.

Similarly, for specificity, as you define it, draw an arrow moving UP the right column, to represent all those without disease with a negative test, over all those without disease.

Have the learners calculate the actual sensitivity and specificity for the example you have chosen. Ask them, given your patient's test result, if they can articulate your patient's probability of disease with these numbers. We cannot!

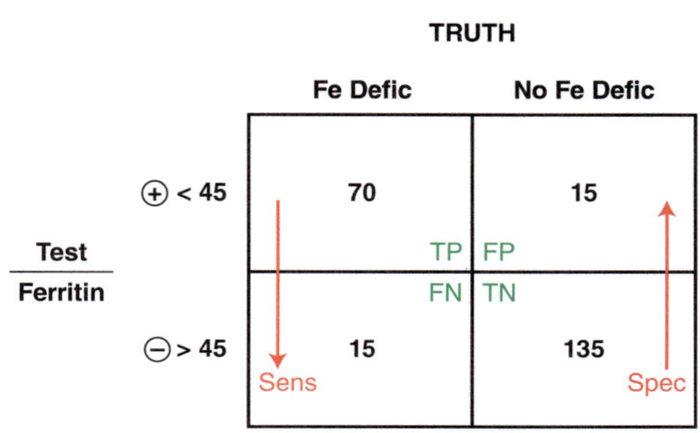

Fig. 7.3 Visual depiction of sensitivity and specificity

Likelihood Ratios: Introduction to the Concept

Likelihood ratios allow us to move from the patient's pre-test probability of disease, what we thought before we ordered the test, to their post-test probability of disease, how likely disease is now, given our test result.

Likelihood ratios can be tricky to teach, but with a few core memory and visual aids, the teaching can be extremely effective and learners will leave with tools which reinforce their clinical decision making.

The teaching tools discussed here are also depicted in Video 7.1 *which accompanies this chapter.*

30–60 min:

After the sensitivity and specificity exercise above, ask the learners if they can take a stab at defining likelihood ratios.

A likelihood ratio is a ratio of two likelihoods [7]! What goes on top, and what goes on the bottom? We suggest having learners remember the formula in terms of "WITH disease over WITHOUT disease". This will always be true, in every likelihood ratio. You can start writing the ratio on the board in this way—if the likelihood ratio is the ratio of two likelihoods, the one on top involves patients WITH disease and the one on the bottom involves patients WITHOUT disease.

Continue on the board with the definition of a "positive" likelihood ratio as you build it together. Move the group to the following definition: (+) LR = Proportion of patients WITH disease with a positive test result/proportion of patients WITHOUT disease with a positive test result, as in Fig. 7.4.

Move back to the 2 × 2 table you drew previously, with the contrasting arrows to signify sensitivity and specificity schematically. Ask the group, what is "the proportion of patients WITH disease with a positive test"? Well, it's the same as the sensitivity! We just defined that! What is "the proportion of patients WITHOUT disease with POSITIVE test"? Ah, now we need to flip over specificity—we can draw a dotted line in the same contrasting color, moving DOWN the WITHOUT DISEASE column of our 2 × 2 table, to represent our specificity flipped over, as in Fig. 7.5. Write on the board, (+) LR = sensitivity/1-specificity.

Now, tackle a "negative" likelihood ratio. The converse of what we just demonstrated will come through. Ask the group to try to define it. Move the group towards the following definition: (−) LR = Proportion of patients WITH disease with a NEGATIVE test/proportion of patients WITHOUT disease with a NEGATIVE test.

Move to the 2 × 2 table again, and visually demonstrate that, the (−) LR = 1-sensitivity/specificity.

Calculate the likelihood ratios for the data you have chosen, from the sensitivity and specificity.

Remind the group that LRs are ALWAYS "with disease" over "without disease". You might hold your hands in the air to represent a ratio or draw a large ratio on the board that simply states "with" over "without". The likelihood ratio can only be one of three things: Greater than 1, less than 1, or 1 [7]. "If you see a positive test result, you sure hope it happens more often in patients WITH disease! A good positive likelihood ratio is a BIG number!" "If you see a negative test result, you sure hope it happens more often in patients WITHOUT disease! A good negative likelihood ratio is a SMALL number!" Learners will often ask 'how big' or 'how small' does it need to be. It's ok to give "10" and "0.10" as examples, but emphasize that the important thing is how the likelihood ratios play out when applied to pre-test probability, which comes next. And, of course, what does it mean when the likelihood ratio is 1? That result does not discriminate between those with and without disease, at all!!

Fig. 7.4 Likelihood ratio definition

$$\oplus \text{ LR} = \frac{\text{Proportion WITH DISEASE} \oplus \text{ test}}{\text{Proportion WITHOUT DISEASE} \oplus \text{ test}} = \frac{\text{Sens}}{\text{1-spec}}$$

$$\ominus \text{ LR} = \frac{\text{Proportion WITH DISEASE} \ominus \text{ test}}{\text{Proportion WITHOUT DISEASE} \ominus \text{ test}} = \frac{\text{1-Sens}}{\text{spec}}$$

Fig. 7.5 Likelihood ratio visual depiction

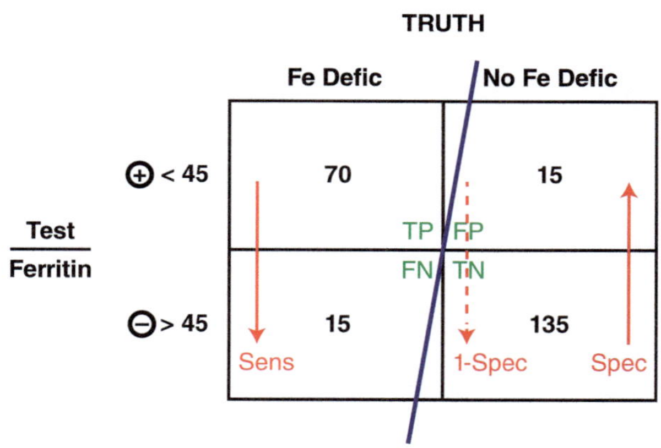

Likelihood Ratios: Applying Them to Patient Care

10–15 min:

Once the learner has a clinical scenario in hand, with a pre-test probability estimate and a likelihood ratio associated with a test result, bring out the Fagan Nomogram and use it to move to post-test probability. Instruct learners on how to use the Nomogram, utilizing photocopied versions on paper so that they can interact with it directly. After they arrive at a post-test probability, ask them what the post-test probability needs to be in order to take the next clinical step. This will vary by clinical condition! It may be helpful to provide extreme and almost ridiculous examples, of two different conditions where the post-test probability needed to take action are very different—for instance, allergic rhinitis vs. cancer.

With the nomogram in front of them, this is an ideal time to demonstrate how the interpretation of a test result varies widely depending on the pre-test probability. Have the group change the pre-test probability for the scenario they just used to something very, very low. Move through the SAME likelihood ratio. What happens? The post-test probability is not nearly as impressive. Thus, you have demonstrated that the pre-test probability is actually far more important than the test itself. Continue to play with the nomogram using hypothetical situations: a very very strong positive test in a very low pretest probability population still does not make the diagnosis likely, and, conversely, a very very strong negative test in a high pre-test probability population does not lessen the chance of disease very much. In general medicine learners, it is useful to talk about a patient scenario that is high pre-test probability (>90%) for acute coronary syndrome. Would a negative stress test change your plan? No, your suspicion would remain high and you would take that patient to the cath lab.

15 min:

If you have more time and are so inclined, you might also teach the math behind the nomogram. You can have learners convert their pre-test probability to a pre-test odds, multiply by the LR, and then arrive at a post-test odds. Converting that back to post-test probability will arrive at the same answer as the nomogram provided.

Likelihood Ratios: Calculating Them for Different Levels of a Test

The beauty of likelihood ratios is that they can be calculated for multiple levels of the test, they need not be restricted to dichotomous test results. Here we will describe a teaching session which is adapted from the work of Richardson et al. [7] and utilizes a 1990 paper on the accuracy of ferritin for diagnosing iron deficiency in the elderly [6].

15–30 min:

Following the three lessons above, prepare the dry erase board with a table 4 columns wide and 7 rows long. Column #1 is "ferritin", column #2 is "iron deficiency", column #3 is "no iron deficiency", and leave column #4 blank for now so that learners don't immediately guess where you're headed, as depicted in Fig. 7.6. Worksheets 7.3 and 7.4 are provided in the Appendix as guides as well.

For the "ferritin" column, fill in the following values: >100, 45–100, 18–45, <18, and total.

In the "iron deficiency" and "no iron deficiency" columns, fill in the raw numbers from Table 3 [6] in Worksheets 7.3. Under "the iron deficiency article", it would be 8, 7, 23, 47 and in the "no iron deficiency" it would be 108, 27, 13, 2. The totals for the columns are 85 and 150, respectively.

Ask the group, "Among patients with iron deficiency, what proportion had a ferritin greater than 100?". The group will say 8/85. Then ask "among patients with iron deficiency, what proportion had a ferritin of 45–100?". The group will say 7/85, and so on—start filling in the table on both columns with these proportions, using 150 as the total on the no iron deficiency side, and having the learners get out their calculators to help you.

Now, unveil column #4 as "Likelihood Ratio". Ask the group, what is the likelihood ratio at a ferritin of 100? Often, a learner will be tempted to say it in terms of the sensitivity/1-specificity. Remind them that it's simply WITH over WITHOUT. As they look at the table you created together, it will become evident that the numbers are right in front of them—they need only make a ratio between the "iron deficiency" column and "no iron deficiency" column. Have them fill in the math in column #4 with these ratios, as in Fig. 7.7.

Have learners look at the list of Likelihood Ratios you've generated. What do they notice? The ratios move from below 1 to above 1. There seems to be an inflection point at 45. In the prior exercise, we had collapsed the values of this table using 45 as our cutoff. It was indeed the best cutoff, if we force ourselves to pick one! But, importantly, we gain more information from leaving the levels of the test intact. In fact, where we found a LR of 8 for a positive test result previously, it turns out the LR for a ferritin of 18–45 is only 3, substantially lower.

Recap by telling the group that, while you started this series of lessons by basing your calculations in sensitivity and specificity, these constructs are only relevant when the test results are dichotomous. At multiple levels of the test, we get more information, and we can't calculate sensitivities and specificities at all. In fact, we never really need them. All we need is the ratio of the proportion of patients with that test result WITH disease over WITHOUT!!

Fig. 7.6 Likelihood ratios at different levels of a test, part I

Ferritin	FeDefic	NO FeDefic
>100	$\frac{8}{85}$	$\frac{108}{150}$
45 – 100	$\frac{7}{85}$	$\frac{27}{150}$
18 – 45	$\frac{23}{85}$	$\frac{13}{150}$
<18	$\frac{47}{85}$	$\frac{2}{150}$
Total	85	150

Fig. 7.7 Likelihood ratios at different levels of a test, part II

Ferritin	FeDefic	ϕ	LR
>100	$\frac{8}{85} = .09$	$\frac{108}{150} = .72$	$\frac{.09}{.72} = 0.125$
45 – 100	$\frac{7}{85} = .08$	$\frac{27}{150} = .18$	$\frac{.08}{.18} = 0.44$
18 – 45	$\frac{23}{85} = .27$	$\frac{13}{150} = .08$	$\frac{.27}{.08} = 3$
<18	$\frac{47}{85} = 55.3$	$\frac{2}{150} = 1.33$	$\frac{55.3}{1.33} = 42$
Total	85	150	

Appendix

Worksheet 7.0—Critical appraisal of diagnosis studies

Diagnostic testing critical appraisal worksheet

Assessing the risk of bias	
Do the patients studied represent the population of patients in whom the test will be used, with a similar risk for the disorder?	
Was a reliable gold standard used as a comparator,	
Were the results of the test and the gold standard independent of one another?	
Did all of the patients studied receive both the test and the gold standard?	
Assessing the results	
Were likelihood ratios calculated, or can they be derived from the data provided? Were confidence intervals reported?	
Applying the results	
Is the test feasible to employ in my setting?	
Does this test help to make diagnostic decisions in my patient population?	

Worksheet 7.1—Diagnosis exercise, blank

Diagnostic Testing Worksheet

The Case: [Set up a case involving a patient represented within your article of interest, where there is diagnostic uncertainty]

Question 1: What is your pretest probability (prevalence) of the condition in your patient? How do you establish this?

The Task: Based on the article provided, construct the following 2x2 table, making clear the definition of positive and negative tests if needed.

	Disease present	Disease absent
Test Pos		
Test Neg		

Calculations:

Sensitivity = ______________________________

Specificity = ______________________________

Positive Likelihood Ratio = ____________________

Negative Likelihood Ratio = ___________________

Question 2: Based on the likelihood ratio you calculated, and using the nomogram provided, what is the post-test probability of the condition of interest?

Bonus Question: Describe positive predictive value and discuss why it changes as prevalence changes. Use the nomogram to demonstrate!

Worksheet 7.2—Diagnosis exercise, iron deficiency example

Diagnostic Testing Worksheet

Using "Diagnosing Iron Deficiency Anemia in the Elderly", Guyatt et al. 1990, Am J Med vol 88, p.205-209

The Case: You are treating a 75 year old man in the CCU post-MI. You note a mild anemia on routine labs, with a Hct of 33 and an MCV of 89. There is no clinically evident bleeding. You want to know if he has iron deficiency, and you order some labs – the ferritin is 39, and is listed in the normal range of values on the lab report.

Question 1: What is your pretest probability (prevalence) of iron deficiency anemia in this patient?

The Task: Based on the article you have read, construct the following 2x2 table, using a cutoff of ferritin below 45 as positive, and above 45 as negative. (where do you find this information in the article?)

	Disease present	Disease absent
Test Pos		
Test Neg		

Calculations:

Sensitivity = ______________________________

Specificity = ______________________________

Positive Likelihood Ratio = ____________________

Negative Likelihood Ratio = ___________________

Question 2: Based on the likelihood ratio you calculated, and using the nomogram in the handout, what is the post-test probability of iron deficiency anemia?

Bonus Question: Describe positive predictive value and discuss why it changes as prevalence changes. Use the nomogram to demonstrate!

Worksheet 7.3—Likelihood ratio exercise, iron deficiency, blank

Liklihood Ratios Can be Calculated for Multiple Levels of a Test

This exercise is based on the article, "Diagnosing Iron Deficiency Anemia in the Elderly", Guyatt et al. 1990, Am J Med vol 88, p. 205-209. This one of the best articles availble for teaching how to calculate the likelihood ratio for mutiple levels of a test.

The Task: Based on the article provided, construct the following 2x2 table

	Iron Deficiency present	Iron Deficiency absent
Ferritin >100		
Ferritin 45-100		
Ferritin 18-45		
Ferritin <18		
Total		

Now, Add in another column for Likelihood Ratio:

	Iron Deficiency present	Iron Deficiency absent	Likelihood Ratio
Ferritin >100			
Ferritin 45-100			
Ferritin 18-45			
Ferritin <18			
Total			

How do you calculate the Likelihood Ratio at each level of the test?

What do you notice about the Likelihood Ratios?

Worksheet 7.4—Likelihood ratio exercise, iron deficiency, answers

Liklihood Ratios Can be Calculated for Multiple Levels of a Test

This exercise is based on the article,"Diagnosing Iron Deficiency Anemia in the Elderly", Guyatt et al. 1990, Am J Med vol 88, p.205-209. This is one of the best articles available for teaching how to calculate the likelihood ratio for multiple levels of a test.

The Task: Based on the article provided, construct the following 2x2 table

	Iron Deficiency present	Iron Deficiency absent
Ferritin >100	8	108
Ferritin 45-100	7	27
Ferritin 18-45	23	13
Ferritin <18	47	2
Total	85	150

Now, Add in another column for Likelihood Ratio:

	Iron Deficiency present	Iron Deficiency absent	Likelihood Ratio
Ferritin >100	8/85 = .09	108/150 = .72	.09/.72 = **0.13**
Ferritin 45-100	7/85 = .08	27/150 = .18	.08/.18 = **0.46**
Ferritin 18-45	23/85 = .27	13/150 = .09	.27/.09 = **3**
Ferritin <18	47/85 = .553	2/150 = .013	.553/.013 = **42**
Total	85	150	

How do you calculate the Likelihood Ratio at each level of the test?

It is simply the proportion of people WITH disease with that test result divided by the proportion of people WITHOUT disease with that test result!

What do you notice about the Likelihood Ratios? Where is the inflection point, where the LR goes from negative to positive?

As the Ferritin gets lower, the likelihood ratio gets bigger. The inflection point is at a ferritin of 45. It seems that a Ferritin lower than 18 is a much stronger positive test than a ferritin of 30!

References

1. Rahnsohoff DF, Feinstein AR. Problems of spectrum and bias in evaluating the efficacy of diagnostic tests. N Engl J Med. 1978;299(17):926–30.
2. Montori VM, Wyer P, et al. Tips for learners of evidence-based medicine: 5. The effect of spectrum of disease on the performance of diagnostic tests. CMAJ. 2005;173(4):385–90.
3. Furukawa TA, Straus SE, et al. Diagnostic tests. In: Guyatt G, Rennie D, Meade MO, Cook DJ, editors. User's guides to the medical literature: a manual for evidence based clinical practice. 3rd ed. Sherborn: JAMAevidence; 2015.
4. Buchsbaum DG, Buchanan RG, et al. Screening for alcohol abuse using CAGE scores and likelihood ratios. Ann Intern Med. 1991;115(10):774–7.
5. Fagan TJ. Nomogram for Bayes' theorem. N Engl J Med. 1975;293(5):257.
6. Guyatt GH, Patterson C, et al. Diagnosis of iron-deficiency anemia in the elderly. Am J Med. 1990;88:205–9.
7. Richardson WS, Wilson MC, et al. Tips for teachers of evidence-based medicine: making sense of diagnostic test results using likelihood ratios. J Gen Intern Med. 2007;23(1):87–92.

Screening

8

Daniella A. Zipkin and Matthew Tuck

Guide for the Teacher

Screening is not typically a separate, core topic in evidence based medicine curricula, yet it tends to be widely misunderstood and we believe it deserves special attention. Screening is a type of intervention, and therefore shares core features regarding assessing validity and understanding the numeric presentation of results with Therapy. The randomized controlled trial is the ideal study design to assess the impact of screening. While screening requires a diagnostic test as a tool, the topic is not about the accuracy or validity of diagnostic tests, which is covered elsewhere (see Chap. 7). Instead, we apply a diagnostic tool as an intervention to a population of asymptomatic persons in an effort to diagnose conditions earlier and to improve mortality or other important clinical outcomes. Many of us grew up with the adage "an ounce of prevention is worth a pound of cure." It seems intuitive that screening would always be beneficial, so some may wonder why we study it at all. However, all

Supplementary Information The online version contains supplementary material available at [https://doi.org/10.1007/978-3-031-11174-7_8].

D. A. Zipkin (✉)
Department of Medicine, Duke University Health System,
Duke University School of Medicine, Durham, NC, USA
e-mail: daniella.zipkin@duke.edu

M. Tuck
Department of Medicine, Veterans Affairs Medical Center, Medical Service,
George Washington University, Washington, DC, USA
e-mail: Matthew.Tuck@va.gov

D. A. Zipkin (ed.), *Teaching Evidence-Based Medicine*,
https://doi.org/10.1007/978-3-031-11174-7_8

interventions carry potential harms and costs and if we are to adopt screening widely, we want to ensure that there is a mortality benefit compared to not screening.

On the surface it may seem that the topic of screening is most important for primary care specialties such as pediatrics, family medicine, obstetrics and gynecology, and general internal medicine. However, we believe that the impact is much broader. Decisions about screening involve radiologists, oncologists, subspecialists of medicine, general surgeons, breast surgeons, urologists, and so on. For this reason, we strongly recommend leaving space to discuss screening in your evidence-based medicine curriculum, regardless of your clinical audience. The topic can be covered in as little as 30 min or for as long as you need. At the minimum, we recommend ensuring that your learners can articulate the critical difference between *survival* and *mortality*, and define *lead time bias*.

Introduction

The objective of screening is the early detection of pre-symptomatic disease and subsequent management at a stage of disease that presumably carries lower morbidity and mortality. While it may seem intuitive to both health care providers and lay persons that early detection would always be a good idea, that is not, in fact, always the case. The decision to implement screening is an intervention like any other, and needs to stand up to scrutiny in the assessment of its benefits and harms.

Certain assumptions need to be true when we employ a test in screening: (1) the prevalence of the condition in the population is high enough to make screening feasible, (2) the biologic onset of disease precedes symptoms, (3) the correct test can detect disease at this early point, and (4) identifying disease at an earlier time point leads to therapy which is more effective than later. *Screening is an intervention*, one which *employs* a diagnostic test. Studies of screening, therefore, should meet the criteria for any study of an *intervention*—randomization into screened and non-screened groups discussed below (Box 8.1) [1]. Cohort and cross-sectional studies are inadequate in answering screening questions because they are vulnerable to several important biases.

Box 8.1 Minimizing Bias in Studies of Screening

- Screening recommendations should be based upon randomized controlled trials of screening compared to no screening in asymptomatic people whenever possible.
- Methodologic criteria for randomized trials should be followed, see Chap. 4.

Sources of Bias in Studies of Screening

Lead Time Bias

Survival is defined as the time from diagnosis until death or recurrence as shown schematically in Fig 8.1. *Early diagnosis will always appear to improve survival, even when therapy does not change mortality*. Because survival is defined as the time from diagnosis to death or recurrence, increasing survival may mean subjects have simply known about the disease longer, not actually lived longer [2]. Early diagnosis shifts the time point for calculating the survival estimate forward. This is why disease-specific *mortality* is a more clinically important outcome than *survival*. How do we address the possibility of lead time bias? *Do a randomized trial!* A randomized trial can eliminate lead time bias by gathering subjects at the same time point, randomizing some to screening and some to no screening, then following forward to determine the mortality benefit associated with the screening arm—irrespective of survival. Fig 8.2 demonstrates schematically how Lead Time Bias can be become evident when a randomized trial is conducted. Lead Time Bias visual aids are also depicted in the TEACH IT section below and in Video 8.1.

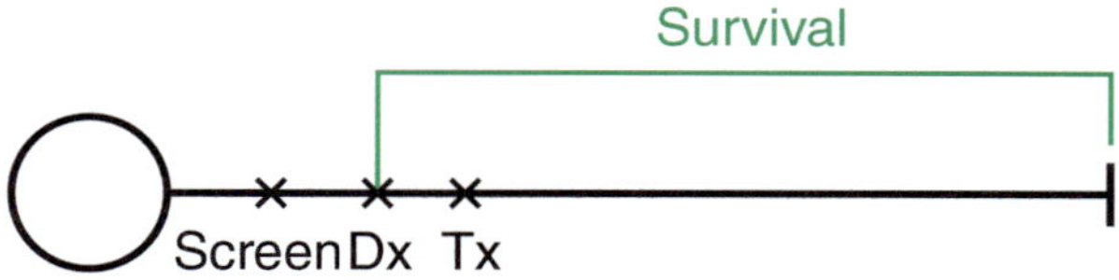

Fig. 8.1 Lead time bias, part I. Survival is defined as time from diagnosis until death or recurrence. If we have a single cohort and no comparison group, early detection will always improve survival, because it is defined by the time of diagnosis. Without a comparison group, we cannot know whether or not this group has better mortality than an un-screened group

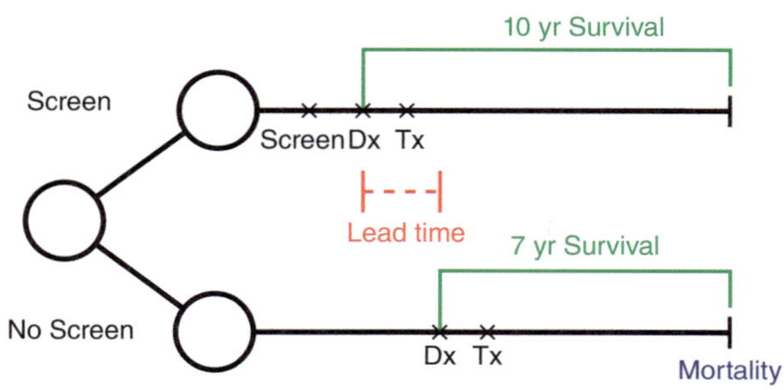

Fig. 8.2 Lead time bias, part II. If death rates are similar at the end of the study, *survival* may be longer in the screened group, but *mortality* is not improved, as demonstrated in this graphic. *Lead time* represents the additional time that the screened group was aware of the diagnosis, without a benefit in mortality

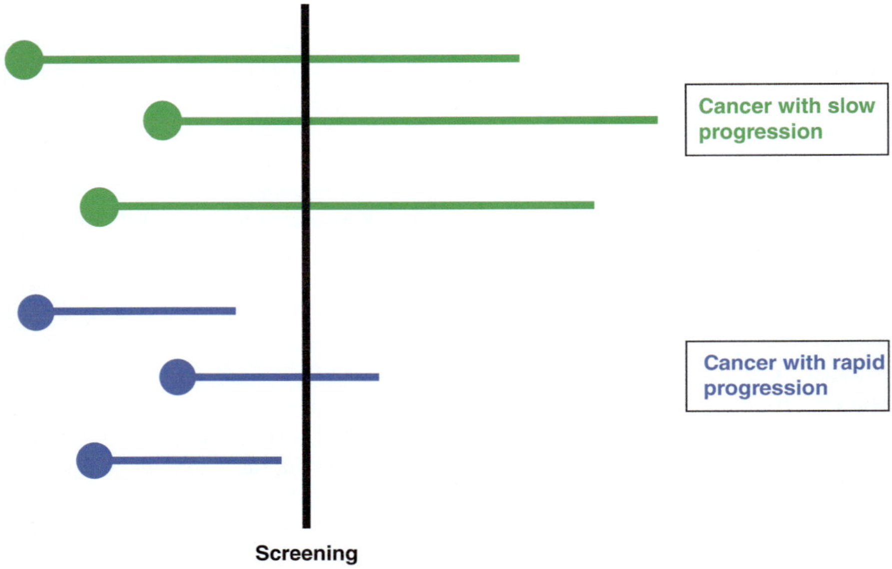

Fig. 8.3 Length time bias. Screening will find more people living with the slowly progressive cancer. Without a comparison group, one might attribute those patients doing well to the screening itself. In this schematic diagram, circles represent disease onset and horizontal lines indicate survival

Length Time Bias

Slowly progressive diseases are easier to detect than faster ones because they are more prevalent at any given point in time. Therefore, people with diseases found more easily through screening may appear to live longer, as depicted in Fig. 8.3. Imagine the differences between pancreatic cancer with its rapid mortality rate, and prostate cancer where people can do well for many years. Do patients with prostate cancer survive longer because they were screened, or because their cancer is more indolent? It is easy to fall into the trap of attributing improved survival to the screening in a cohort design, but it may in fact be due to the prognosis of the disease. *How do we fix length time bias? Do a randomized trial*, to eliminate the impact of length of time on your findings, and even out confounding variables between the groups. A length time bias visual aid is also depicted in Video 8.1.

Volunteerism Bias

People who volunteer for screening studies may be more concerned about their health, and therefore healthier than non-volunteers. Studies regarding screening may not represent outcomes in the general population. How do we fix volunteerism bias? Well, you really cannot; we have to accept that trial results never fully approximate the real world.

When the benefits of screening appear strong and consistent and drawbacks are minimal, widespread screening may be implemented based on observational data alone, as is the case with cervical cancer screening. A randomized controlled trial of Pap screening for cervical cancer has never been done, because population-wide reduction in rates of cancer after screening was implemented were so compelling. More often, however, the benefits and risks of screening are more closely aligned, and randomized trial data is needed.

The results of a screening trial will often be presented as *absolute risk reduction* and *relative risk reduction*. Please refer to Chapter 4 Therapy for a discussion of these concepts. *Number needed to screen* can be calculated in the same way as number needed to treat.

Balancing Benefits and Harms in Screening

In assessing the benefits of screening, it is important to note which *outcomes* were chosen. *Mortality* reduction is the ultimate goal. Cause-specific mortality, or mortality specifically related to the condition in question, is the most important outcome. If the burden caused by the disease is high, then lowering cause-specific mortality may also impact overall mortality, or death due to any cause. Other outcomes may include health related quality of life and "intangibles" such as reassurance, or piece of mind.

The risks of screening may include anxiety, complications from pursuit of a diagnosis, side effects of treatment, adverse effects of labeling a patient with a diagnosis, and costs of work-up and therapy. Some clinical scenarios, such as breast cancer screening and prostate cancer screening, lend themselves well to a discussion of benefit vs harm of screening. Benefits and harms can be quantified and directly compared using absolute risk reduction and absolute risk increase. For instance, with breast cancer, the estimated reduction in breast cancer mortality for an average risk woman can be compared to the risk of anxiety and distress with false positives, lumpectomy and mastectomy rates, and the cost and burden of actually having mammograms performed.

TEACH IT!!

Lead Time Bias

Visual aids for this teaching segment are also depicted in Video 8.1

15 min:

Start with a cohort diagram on the board, like Fig. 8.1: A circle at the start of the study, a horizontal line extending to the right, and then a vertical line at the endpoint of the study. Mark an "X" along the line near the start, and label it "screen". Draw an "X" immediately to the right of the screen point and label it "diagnosis". Draw a bracket from your "diagnosis" point to the endpoint of the cohort. Ask the group what this interval is called. The answer is SURVIVAL. We define survival from the point of diagnosis to either death or recurrence, however we define it.

Now ask the group—if the survival we measure in the cohort is on average 10 years, but historically survival from this condition has averaged 7 years, have we improved survival with screening? The answer is YES—survival is indeed increased, because we define survival as the time from diagnosis to death or recurrence. Now ask the group, have we improved mortality? The answer is WE DON'T KNOW. It is not possible to know that from this design!

Draw a second cohort diagram beneath the first one, and then connect them via a larger circle to the left of the starting point, like Fig. 8.2. You've drawn a randomized controlled trial! The arm you already indicated with screening is the screening arm, and the new arm does not receive screening. Mark a point of diagnosis some time later than the first group's point of diagnosis, because on average diagnoses will be made later when we don't screen, but extend the cohort lines to the same endpoint as the top line. Draw a bracket for the second arm from diagnosis to the endpoint of that arm.

Now ask the group, has survival increased in the screening group? YES. Has mortality improved in the screening group? No, overall mortality is the same, after sufficient time passes. That is LEAD TIME BIAS. Draw a bracket in a contrasting color between the two arms, stretching from the diagnosis of the first arm to the diagnosis of the second arm. This is the degree of LEAD TIME achieved by screening. Screening has allowed people to know about their disease longer, without actually improving mortality.

Lead time bias is the reason we must do randomized controlled trials of screening tests. Screening will ALWAYS improve survival, because of how we define survival. To assess mortality, we need an RCT.

30 min:

Gather sample studies of screening modalities relevant to your learners. There are metanalyses of randomized controlled trials for breast cancer screening and prostate cancer screening. There are large randomized trials on the topics of colon cancer screening and ovarian cancer screening. Review selected abstracts or full papers with your learners. Ask them if the study design is appropriate for the question and if it effectively manages the possibility of lead time bias. Then, review the results, and express them in terms of absolute reductions in risk, number needed to screen, or icon arrays. This exercise frames the magnitude of impact of screening for learners.

10 min/on the fly:

In the clinical context, resources exist to help get to screening recommendations quickly. These include:

US Preventive Services Task Force recommendations, available online.
Agency for Healthcare Research and Quality guideline reports.
Quick glance at a Cochrane review abstract summary.

References

1. McCaffery KJ, Jacklyn GL, Barratt A, Brodersen J, Glasziou P, Carter SM, Hicks NR, Howard K, Irwig L, editors. Recommendations about screening. In: Users' guides to the medical literature: a manual for evidence-based clinical practice. 3rd ed. Washington, DC: American Medical Association; 2015.
2. Zelen M, Feinleib M. On the theory of screening for chronic diseases. Biometrika. 1969;56(3):601–14.

Prognosis

9

Daniella A. Zipkin and Jeffrey Kushinka

Guide for the Teacher
Prognosis refers to survival and expected disease course and is sometimes included as a core content section in evidence-based medicine curricula. Prognosis is an excellent place to expand on issues affecting cohort studies as well as incorporate Kaplan–Meier curves and hazard ratios. It is particularly relevant for fields such as oncology, where clinical cure is not always feasible, so maximizing disease-free survival is more relevant. Prognosis can also prompt discussions about the creation and use of clinical prediction rules.

Introduction

Prognosis refers to the possible outcomes of a disease and the frequency with which they can be expected to occur. Because assessing prognosis requires that groups of patients similar to your patient are followed over time, the best study design within which to assess prognosis is a *cohort* study, or within an arm of a *randomized controlled trial.*

D. A. Zipkin (✉)
Department of Medicine, Duke University Health System,
Duke University School of Medicine, Durham, NC, USA
e-mail: daniella.zipkin@duke.edu

J. Kushinka
Department of Internal Medicine, Virginia Commonwealth University School of Medicine,
Richmond, VA, USA
e-mail: Jeffrey.kushinka@vcuhealth.org

D. A. Zipkin (ed.), *Teaching Evidence-Based Medicine*,
https://doi.org/10.1007/978-3-031-11174-7_9

Sources of Bias in Studies of Prognosis

It is important to determine if the sample of study patients is representative of our patient, because systematic differences between the populations will lead to biased estimates of prognosis [1]. One of the most common ways in which study patients may differ from the individual patient in front of us involves *referral-filter bias*. Patients who have been referred to specialists have different risk factors and do not represent the entire group of patients with the issue of interest, therefore their prognosis may differ greatly from our patient's prognosis.

In addition, because prognosis depends on the natural history of disease, which incorporates disease severity and the passage of time, it is important to capture patients at a similar point in their course of disease, and this should be consistent across the group [1]. If we group patients at very different points in the course of disease, prognostic estimates will be unreliable. This is why we need an *inception cohort*—patients identified at a sufficiently early and uniform point in their disease, such that those who succumb or completely recover will be included with those whose disease persists, and we can estimate the probability of various outcomes. Groups should also be homogeneous with respect to other important prognostic factors. If they are not, i.e., if there are important factors that vary among the subjects, the study should report the statistical techniques used to *adjust* for those variables. This process is the same as the process discussed in Chap. 6.

Follow-up is extremely important when prognosis is being assessed [1]. Sufficient time must pass to allow for various disease outcomes to occur. Investigators must minimize loss to follow-up, though precisely how much loss to follow-up is too much is subject to debate. A useful approach is to compare those lost to follow-up with the proportion of patients who developed an outcome. Would the results change significantly if all of those lost to follow-up had developed the outcome? If they had not? If so, then the loss to follow-up may alter your findings to an unacceptable degree.

In addition, investigators must be consistent in applying objective outcome assessments to all participants. If some outcomes are missed, estimates or prognosis will be inaccurate. If we are more likely to miss outcomes in groups with certain prognostic factors compared to those without the prognostic factors, our estimates will also be biased (Box 9.1).

Box 9.1 Managing Sources of Bias in Studies of Prognosis

- Make sure the sample being studied matches your patient population in terms of risk factors for disease progression.
- Make sure the sample consists of patients at a uniform point in the disease process.
- Follow-up should be sufficient to allow for a wide range of potential outcomes to occur, and the outcome assessments should be clear and applied uniformly to the whole sample.

Clinical Prediction Rules

Clinical prediction rules can help take some uncertainty out of prognosis and aid decision making. They are statistically derived sets of clinical variables from the history, physical exam, and diagnostic tests which, when combined, generate a probability of a particular diagnosis or prognosis. These rules are created from cohorts of patients. A *derivation cohort* serves as the initial data is assessed, with statistical modeling of the predictive ability of various clinical factors. Once derived, the rule should then be applied to a separate *validation cohort* to ensure it performs as expected. Derivation and validation cohorts should be large and broad enough to represent a wide spectrum of prognoses. The error rate which occurs in this process of testing a rule in a validation cohort is known as the mis-classification rate, or how many patients would have been mis-classified into the wrong prognosis by the rule, in comparison with observed outcomes.

Sources of bias in clinical prediction rule development include poorly defined outcome events, poorly defined predictive findings, and failure to blind those who define the predictors or the outcomes [2]. Predictors and outcomes must be clearly defined, objective and reproducibly assessed. Also, outcome assessment should be blinded—or performed without knowledge of the predictor variables—to avoid the natural tendency to bias observers toward a conclusion based on other data. A validated rule is applicable to clinical practice when the predicted outcomes are pertinent and the predictors are feasible and relevant [2]. Clinical prediction rules should be applied to the same general population in which they were developed. Many validated clinical prediction rules are in common use to assist clinicians with decision making on a whole range of situations, from myocardial infarction to pulmonary embolism to severity of head injury or abdominal pain in children to risk of morbidity from surgeries.

TEACH IT!!

Inception Cohort

5–10 min:

Draw a series of "cohort lines" to represent different patients with a disease course on the board, originating with a circle, moving forward in time as a line, and ending with a vertical line. Scatter them about the board such that the lines begin in different positions along an x axis, and have different lengths. In a contrasting color, slice through all of your disease course lines with a vertical line at a random point. Ask the learners what would happen if you gathered all of those patients together at that time, and followed them forward to learn something about disease prognosis. Through discussion it will become apparent that if you start following people at different points in the disease course, you will get unclear information about prognosis. Then, imagine pulling all of those lines to the left side so they originate at the zero point of the y axis. Now, observed from the same starting point, they make up an *inception cohort* and can help us determine prognosis.

15–30 min:

Take the concept of inception cohorts and apply it to real data. Prepare one to three abstracts or article ahead of time on an issue of prognosis for a disease relevant to your leaners. Have the learners pore through the methodology, focusing on how patients were recruited into the study, to assess if it was an adequate inception cohort. Were any filters present, such as referral to a specialist? Did patients enter the study at a similar starting point in the course of disease? Was follow-up sufficiently long to have seen relevant outcomes?

Clinical Prediction Rules

15–30 min:

Set up clinical cases in a domain relevant to your setting, where clinical prediction rules can be used. Have learners assess the prognosis of the case on their own first, through group consensus. Then, introduce the clinical prediction rule and see how it honed their estimate. If the estimate didn't change, why not? Were the learners' variables and gut instincts in line with the rule? Great! If there was a change, explore why. What might the rule have included that learners did not? Or, how might our biases affect our perception of risk?

Review the study behind the rule, and ask learners to identify how the variables were defined, how the outcomes were defined, and weather the outcome assessors were blinded. How does the rule stack up?

Prognosis Math

Most studies of prognosis utilize a plot of the proportion of patients experiencing an outcome of interest over a certain period of time, termed a *survival curve*, often more specifically a Kaplan–Meier survival plot [3]. Survival curve plots can visually compare the prognosis of groups with and without a condition. A sample survival curve is shown in Fig. 9.1.

Survival curves can lead to the calculation of *hazard ratios* [4]. While a full review of hazard ratios is beyond the scope of this text, it is useful to convey a working definition which learners can grasp, since many studies in therapy, harm, and prognosis utilize them. The hazard ratio is similar to the risk ratio. The hazard ratio incorporates data from the entire study period by comparing the area under the curves for each group, and calculating the differences in this area over intervals across the study period. Making these intervals infinitesimally small and integrating across the curves generates the hazard ratio. At the end of this process, one can say that the hazard ratio represents "the risk ratio within the next interval of time" between the groups, or "the risk ratio at any point in time along the survival curve". In other words, the hazard ratio tells you, at any point along the curve, what the probability of one group having the outcome would be, compared to the other group, in the next interval of time. See also the discussion of hazard ratios in Chap. 4.

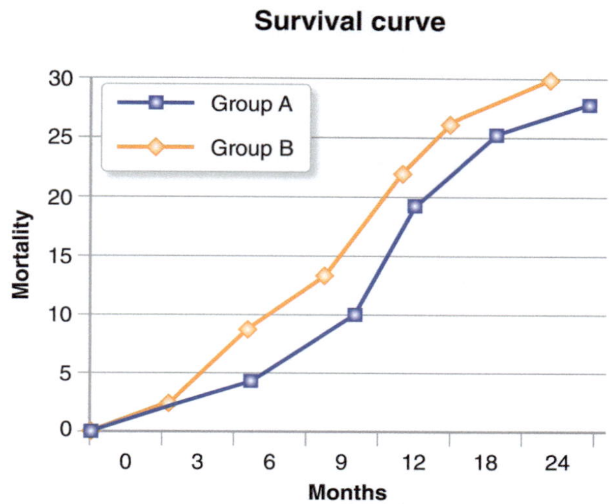

Fig. 9.1 Survival curve. Survival curves track the accrual of events over time, where the starting point is defined in the same way for all participants

TEACH IT!!

Hazard Ratios, a Basic Introduction

This teaching tool is also depicted in Chap. 4, Video 4.1 *which accompanies the Therapy chapter.*

15 min:

Draw the following two diagrams on the board (Fig. 9.2):

Point out that, while the study groups end up at roughly the same difference, one study got there in fairly linear fashion, with that difference being consistent the whole time, and the other study did not—early differences seem to balloon out the curves and create a problem. You'd miss those early deviations if you simply calculated a risk ratio at the end of the study. The Hazard Ratios address the shapes of the curves as they progress.

In a contrasting color, add some vertical line intervals across the curves, like so (Fig. 9.3):

Tell the learners that the Hazard Ratio is derived from the ratio of the area under the top curve over the area under the bottom curve. By integrating across the study period with an infinitesimally small interval, we can derive the Hazard Ratio, which is essentially equivalent to "the risk ratio at any point in time in the study".

Conclude by assuring learners that when they see a Hazard Ratio, they can interpret it as a more robust risk ratio—one that accounts for the shape of the curve over time.

In teaching Therapy, you may encounter studies which present Hazard Ratios, but you are using them to have learners practice calculating the much simpler risk ratio (see Chap. 4). In these instances, it's worthwhile to compare the simple risk ratio with the hazard ratio, and note that for relatively linear data, they will generally be very similar.

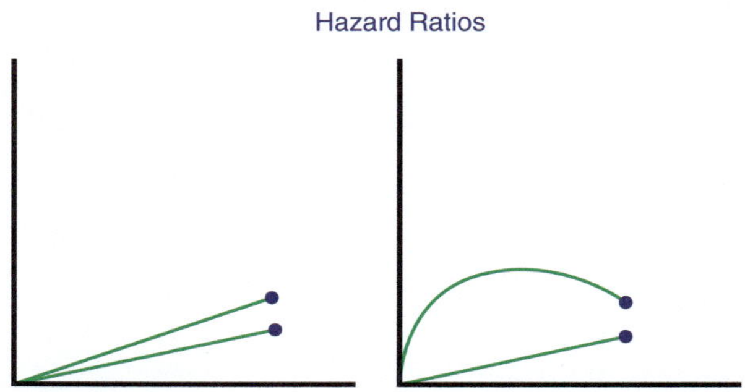

Fig. 9.2 Hazard ratio part I

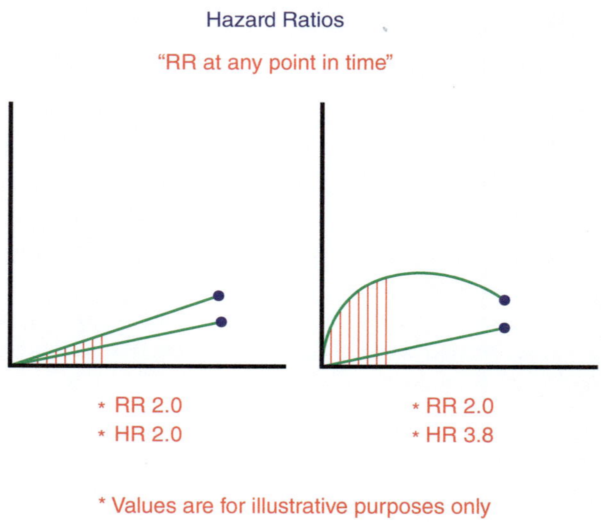

Fig. 9.3 Hazard ratio part II

References

1. Randolph AG, Cook DJ, Guyatt G. Prognosis. In: Guyatt G, Rennie D, Meade MO, Cook DJ, editors. User's guides to the medical literature: a manual for evidence based clinical practice. 3rd ed. Washington, DC: American Medical Association; 2015.
2. Wasson JH, Sox HC, Neff RK, Goldman L. Clinical prediction rules: applications and methodologic standards. N Engl J Med. 1985;313(13):793–9.
3. Rich JT, Neely G, et al. A practical guide to understanding Kaplan-Meier curves. Otolaryngol Head Neck Surg. 2010;143:331–6.
4. Spruance SL, Reid JE, et al. Hazard ratio in clinical trials. Antimicrob Agents Chemother. 2004;48(8):2787–92.

Systematic Reviews and Meta-analysis 10

Daniella A. Zipkin and Megan von Isenburg

Guide for the Teacher

Teaching about systematic reviews is a critical part of any evidence-based medicine curriculum. The synthesis of evidence serves an important purpose in the assessment and application of scientific inquiry. Systematic reviews, at their best, can collect relevant small studies on a particular clinical question and uncover an effect that the individual studies may not have been able to see on their own. Equally important is an appreciation of systematic reviews which have methodologic flaws and may miss important effects or draw inaccurate conclusions. The Cochrane collaboration has enumerated clear standards on the conduct of systematic reviews and creates reliable reviews and meta-analyses on a wide variety of treatment questions. They consider their reviews to be applicable for approximately 5 years, at which time they require updating.

Systematic review refers to the process of framing a question and gathering all studies that answer it. Meta-analysis, on the other hand, is the math of combining the numerical results of the studies into a single point estimate. Not all systematic reviews will perform meta-analysis, and not all meta-analyses need to be done from systematic reviews—however, it is recommended!

D. A. Zipkin (✉)
Department of Medicine, Duke University Health System,
Duke University School of Medicine, Durham, NC, USA
e-mail: daniella.zipkin@duke.edu

M. von Isenburg
Medical Center Library, School of Medicine, Duke University, Durham, NC, USA
e-mail: megan.vonisenburg@duke.edu

D. A. Zipkin (ed.), *Teaching Evidence-Based Medicine*,
https://doi.org/10.1007/978-3-031-11174-7_10

Teaching systematic reviews can occur in 1–2 h of small or large group didactic time and should include the following core sections:

Systematic review methodology
Risk of bias in systematic reviews
Clinical heterogeneity
Statistical heterogeneity
Magnitude of the results
Applying the results of systematic reviews to patients

Introduction

Systematic reviews identify studies that address a specific question and evaluate all eligible studies in summarizing a body of research. Systematic reviews use a uniform and rigorous approach to identifying all relevant studies, displaying the results of these studies, and calculating a summary estimate of the overall results when appropriate. A well-done systematic review can improve upon the random error and wide confidence intervals found in individual small studies by combining them and increasing the precision of the findings. Some systematic reviews contain meta-analysis, the statistical procedure that combines data from multiple studies. When this occurs, the systematic review is often called a meta-analysis. Not all systematic reviews need to be meta-analyses. They may synthesize the studies descriptively when the differences between them or the nature of the research make it inappropriate to combine them mathematically.

In a systematic review, the study *population* is the individual studies themselves. The inclusion and exclusion criteria refer to the criteria used to include studies in the review. Ideally, reviews will also include an assessment of the quality of the individual studies. Furthermore, because most reviews are accessing studies published in the medical literature, studies that are missed in the literature become a core issue. There are several reasons why studies may be conducted but not published: authors may choose not to submit to journals because of negative or uninteresting findings, or journals may choose not to publish due to a variety of factors including the journal's impact factor, the journals clinical priorities, or the quality of the methods or writing. Trying to assess "publication bias" statistically, as we review below, is important in evaluating the degree to which this occurred, because it affects the results of any systematic review.

Systematic Review Methodology

Methods of identifying and including studies, abstracting their data, and presenting data should be *uniform, unbiased, and replicable* [1]. Every systematic review should begin with a clear clinical question, and criteria for inclusion and exclusion should be explicitly stated a priori and adhered to in an unbiased fashion. Investigators should be blinded to the data, journal, and authors whenever possible when making decisions for inclusion, to avoid bias. A medical librarian should assist in building a comprehensive search strategy in multiple databases. The search must be thorough and exhaustive. For some reviews, the grey literature (such as conference abstracts, government reports, and other unpublished data) will also be searched. Screening occurs in stages once the literature search is complete: first the *titles and abstracts* are screened for relevant articles, and then the *full texts* of papers are screened for inclusion according to the pre-specified inclusion criteria. This step should ideally occur in *duplicate*, in a blinded fashion, so that authors must reach consensus on which papers are included. Each paper will then be assessed for risk of bias, often using validated tools. Finally, summary estimates of effect are generated.

Systematic Reviews: Risk of Bias in Identifying Studies

We recommend keeping the following criteria in mind as you assess the risk of bias of any systematic review. When assessing whether the review was exhaustive, consider the following points:

- Was the search done in at least three databases?
- Were database-relevant subject headings used, in addition to keywords?
- Is the search reproducible in at least one database? (Typically the PubMed search is shared as a supplement.)
- Were appropriate limits used for study designs appropriate to the question?
- Were unnecessary limits, such as language and date of publication, avoided?

Magnitude of Results and Heterogeneity

Summary estimates of the reported effects (relative risk, odds ratio, etc.), with confidence intervals, may be calculated. This is essentially an average effect weighted by the size of each study and sometimes accounting for other variables. Many meta-analyses will present summary data in the form of a *Forest plot*. A Forest plot is a tree-like format for representing the effect size and confidence intervals of multiple studies all at once, such that the overall effect can be seen at-a-glance. See the example shown in Fig. 10.1, modeled after a meta-analysis of intra-articular hyaluronic acid in the treatment of knee osteoarthritis [2]:

Combining the results of different studies is only appropriate if they are similar with respect to design, population, intervention, outcome, controls, blinding, etc. These factors relate to the degree of *clinical heterogeneity*. Deciding "how similar" is similar enough is sometimes a judgment call when it comes to the populations tested, the interventions chosen, and the outcomes assessed. Basically, we use the "eyeball test"—line up the study details in a chart and decide if grouping them makes clinical sense.

Statistical heterogeneity refers to the degree of statistical variability between studies, depicted in Fig. 10.2. Most meta-analyses will report that a statistical test

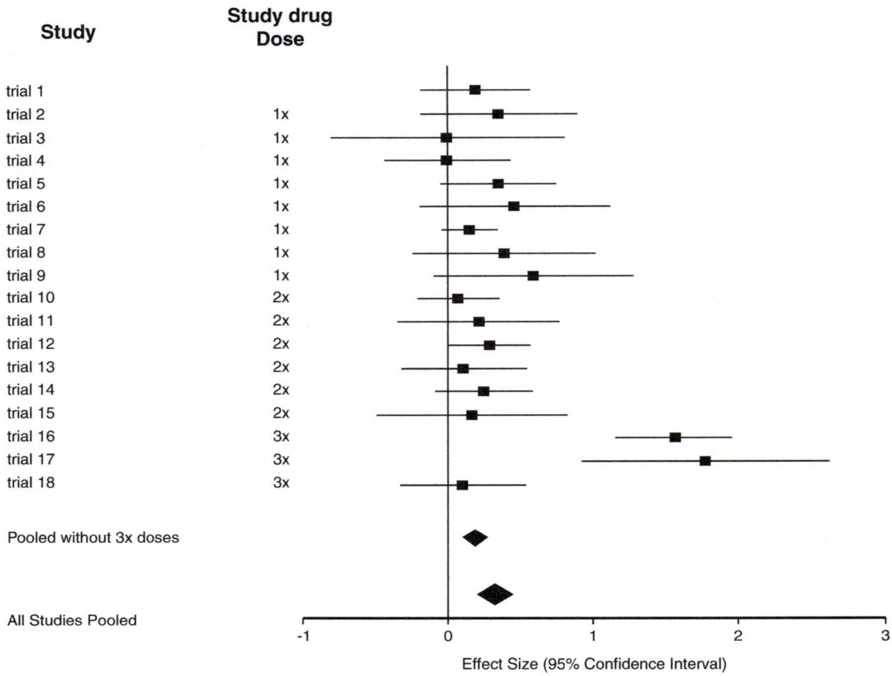

Fig. 10.1 Forest plot example. In this schematic of a Forest plot from a systematic review, note that the effect size of most of the included trials fall between 0 and 1, with many confidence intervals overlapping zero (because zero represents no effect here, they are not statistically significant when taken alone). The overall effect size achieved by combining studies is represented by the larger diamonds at the bottom of the plot and is statistically significant. Thus, taken together, a finding emerges that the individual studies lacked the power to see on their own

Fig. 10.2 Statistical heterogeneity 1. There is more heterogeneity when the confidence intervals of individual studies do not overlap, or are not in the same "neighborhood of truth." In this example, the effect sizes represented by blue squares spend more time in the same neighborhood of truth than the red circles

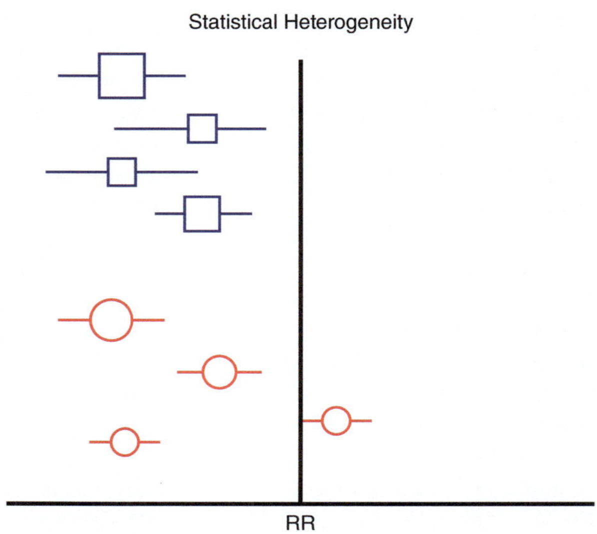

was done to assess for heterogeneity among studies. One commonly used test is the I^2 statistic, which reports statistical heterogeneity on a scale of 0 to 100, with zero meaning no heterogeneity. The I^2 describes the percentage of variability in effect estimates which is due to underlying differences in effect, rather than chance alone, i.e. "less is better." *A rough guide to interpreting the I^2 would be, less than 20% is great, 20–50% is cause for some concern, and over 50% is substantial heterogeneity*. If heterogeneity is present, it must be explained or resolved either by excluding studies with major differences or by stratifying results according to the differences found. If the heterogeneity cannot be resolved, the data should only be combined qualitatively.

Publication bias occurs when published studies are not representative of all of the studies that have been conducted on a topic, usually because positive results tend to be submitted and published more frequently than negative ones. The extent of potential publication bias can be estimated mathematically. Because unpublished studies are more likely to be small and find no effect, a strong correlation between published studies' size and outcome suggests that there is bias. Tests for publication bias are usually presented on a *funnel plot*, which shows sample size vs. outcome measure, as demonstrated in Fig. 10.3. The plot should look like a bell or inverted funnel, with its apex near the summary effect estimate. Imagine, if multiple studies on a similar topic were undertaken, the smallest studies with the greatest random error around the point estimate would fall widely on both sides of the estimate; as studies get larger, they would fall closer to the estimate, forming a sort of "Christmas tree" or inverted funnel. If a funnel plot is lopsided, with the smaller studies (lower down) primarily reporting high effect estimates, publication bias is possible [3]. See, for example, the diagram below:

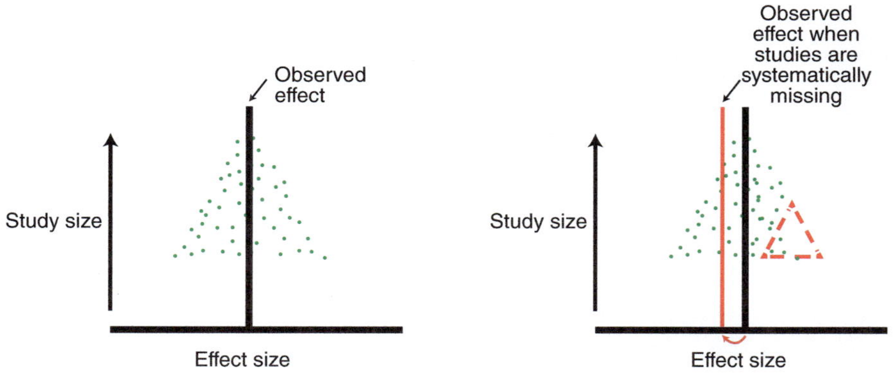

Fig. 10.3 Funnel plot 1. The funnel plot can detect missing studies. Note in this schematic demonstration that the absence of study estimates in the lower right corner might erroneously shift the summative finding to the left

Special Analyses

Subgroup analyses may be done based on data from all or a subset of studies looking at a particular risk group. Subgroup analyses can generate hypotheses regarding the impact of therapies on certain portions of the population. Because sub-groups are smaller portions of their original studies, combining them in a systematic review can make findings more powerful. However, subgroups are often not randomized comparisons (unless the randomization was *stratified* by that subgroup ahead of time), so there may be unmeasured bias on those results. For a more detailed review of subgroup analyses, please see the Chap. 4.

Sensitivity analyses are indicators of how "sensitive" the findings of the meta-analysis are to certain elements of the design of the review or the inclusion of certain studies [1]. Any meta-analysis that includes questionable design decisions or studies which differ in important ways should report a sensitivity analysis as part of its results. In a sensitivity analysis, summary estimates are recalculated after excluding studies with the questionable design element. For example, the findings may be recalculated after excluding studies of lesser quality or particular study populations, to see if it would change the primary results of the meta-analysis.

TEACH IT!!

Systematic Reviews: Risk of Bias

15–30 min:

- Teaching risk of bias in systematic reviews should involve an article reporting a systematic review. If you have time, you can compare and contrast two different articles, one with solid methods, and one with flawed methods. Have learners read through only the methods section of the chosen papers and discuss each point in the recommend list for assessing the risk of bias in systematic reviews. You might tell the learners ahead of time which point they will be responsible for answering, so they will read with that question in mind, if the timing and format allow. Use Worksheet 10.0 in the Appendix for guidance on the full critical appraisal of a systematic review.

TEACH IT!!

Clinical Heterogeneity

10–15 min:

- To briefly address clinical heterogeneity, we recommend conjuring up a fun example to illustrate the concept – perhaps based on your context. For instance, if your session occurs during or after the lunch hour, you might ask a "clinical question" such as "which type of beverage will help learners stay more alert in lectures?" Then, start building an evidence table with the learners' help. Use Worksheets 10.1 and 10.2 in the Appendix as guides. Label the columns Population, Number of subjects, Intervention, Control, Outcome. Label the rows with numbers, or learners' names to keep them engaged. Make up the populations from different schools or specialties (a little friendly competition never hurt anyone!) For instance, team Smith might recruit friends in the surgical residency, and randomize 25 of them to test Red Bull vs. Diet Coke, with the outcome of knot tying time. You get the idea. Fill in the table, while nudging the group towards some similar choices of interventions and outcomes as well as few different ones. Once the table is complete, ask them to use the "eye-ball" test for which of the studies can be combined and which might need to be left out. Ideally, this will lead to a discussion of how different is "too different" to be reliably combined into a summary estimate.

30–60 min:

- If you have more time, expand on the above format with some real articles. Choose a collection of small studies on a particular topic, have the learners' review one article each in teams, and then populate the table based on the methods sections of the papers. Label the columns Population, Number of subjects, Intervention, Control, Outcome. Label the rows with the study author names. After the table is filled in, take a look at it together and decide if the papers are ok to combine. Is there an outlier, or a paper with an intervention or outcome that is too different to be bundled together?

TEACH IT!!

Statistical Heterogeneity

10–15 min:

- Either provide a couple of sample forest plots for learners to examine or draw two simple ones on the board. One should have study effect sizes which are fairly well lined up on one side of the plot, with a little variability in effects but not much, and confidence intervals that all overlap at least a little. The second one, by contrast, should have more variability in the estimates, with some crossing over to the other side, and several with confidence intervals that don't overlap. Have the group discuss—it is easy to see that the plot with a lot of variability has too much statistical heterogeneity, and the wider the numeric differences between the studies the less reliable it is to combine them. The confidence intervals are the key thing here—there needs to be some overlap in the confidence intervals for us to consider combining results. The well-aligned plot would have a LOW I^2 and the scattered plot would have a HIGH I^2, representing a higher degree of variability due to the features of the studies themselves.

TEACH IT!!

Publication Bias

5–10 min:

- It is useful to include a moment talking about publication bias, because funnel plots reinforce the topics of bias and random error in the introductory material to this curriculum.
- Draw a sketch of a funnel plot on the board: A simple line graph with the X axis labeled "RR" (or any measure of effect), and the Y axis labeled "study size" with an arrow going up, so the larger studies are farther up. Draw a "Christmas tree" pattern of dots on the board, representing the increased variability in effect that is found when studies are small, and the tapering upward toward a more reliable effect as studies get larger. This is the ideal situation, when no publication bias exists. Draw a dotted line up through the center of the tree in a contrasting color—this is where a meta-analysis would place a summary effect. (Remind the group that, if you took the axis of the line of effect and tilted it up to point it at the group, the studies would form a "cloud" around the truth similar to that which was mentioned in the bias and random error segment). Now, erase one corner of the base of the tree. Ask the group what would happen if those studies, generally the smaller negative studies, were never published? You would draw a different line of effect—draw a new line, in another color, parallel to the line of effect but slightly over towards the side with the positive studies which did get published. This is the skew in the effect we would find in the case of publication bias. And investigators create funnel plots to guard against this error. Your final diagram should look something like this: Fig. 10.3: Funnel plot 1.

Appendix

Worksheet 10.0—Critical appraisal for systematic reviews

Systematic review critical appraisal worksheet

Assessing the literature search	
Was the literature search exhaustive and performed in all relevant databases?	
Were database-relevant subject headings used, in addition to keywords?	
Were limits used for study designs appropriate to the question?	
Were unnecessary limits, such as language and date of publication, avoided?	
Assessing the inclusion process	
Were inclusion and exclusion criteria explicitly stated?	
Were title and abstract reviews performed in duplicate?	
Were full text reviews for inclusion performed in duplicate?	
Assessing individual study quality	
Was the quality of the individual studies assessed with a reliable instrument?	
Assessing clinical heterogeneity	
Were the populations of the included studies similar?	
Were the interventions of the included studies similar?	
Were the comparison groups of the included studies similar?	
Were the outcomes of the included studies similar	
Assessing statistical heterogeneity	
Assess the Forest plot: Are point estimates similar overall? To what extent do the confidence intervals overlap?	
Are statistical tests which assess between-study variability presented?	
Was the risk of publication bias assessed?	
Applying results	
What is the magnitude and precision of the results?	
Can the findings be applied to my patient population?	

Worksheet 10.1—Systematic review evidence table, blank

Systematic Reviews: Evidence Table Worksheet

Author/year	Population	Number of Subjects	Intervention and control	Outcome Measure(s)	Results:	Study Methodology	Grade of Evidence (A,B,C,D,F) & Why

Worksheet 10.2—Systematic review evidence table, sample

Filling in an evidence table for systematic reviews – example

Author/year	Population	Number of Subjects	Intervention and control	Outcome Measure(s)	Results:	Study Methodology	Grade of Evidence (A,B,C,D,F) & Why
Zipkin, D. 2021* *fake example, article on EBM videos as an intervention for PGY1-2 learners	USA Internal Medicine residents at academic teaching hospitals PGY1-2	498 I: 268 C: 230	I: exposure to EBM videos C: no exposure to EBM videos	Ability to create clinical questions in PICO format Ability to search PubMed Quality of appraisal of selected article	For PICO: 89% For search: ... For appraisal: ...	RCT	B + Randomized Minimal loss to follow up - No concealed allocation No blinding

References

1. Higgins JPT, Green S, editors. Cochrane handbook for systematic reviews of interventions version 5.0.0. London: Cochrane Collaboration; 2008.
2. Lo GH, LaValley M, et al. Intra-articular hyaluronic acid in treatment of knee osteoarthritis: a meta-analysis. JAMA. 2003;290(23):3115–21.
3. Sterne JAC, Sutton AJ, et al. Recommendations for examining and interpreting funnel plot asymmetry in meta-analyses of randomized controlled trials. BMJ. 2011;342:d4002.

Shared Decision Making

11

Zackary D. Berger, Deepa Rani Nandiwada, and Daniella A. Zipkin

Guide for the Teacher

Shared decision making is a bridge from evidence to action. It focuses on the best methods to communicate evidence with the patient in order to support their decision. This topic can stand alone and can also be integrated into each domain of evidence-based medicine as the finale: once learners grasp the core topics, their next challenge will be to learn the best way to bring the information back to their patient to help carry out their preferences.

What follows is a brief review of foundational concepts in shared decision making as well as one suggestion for teaching the topic. We also provide case vignettes applicable to several of our core content chapters illustrating how shared decision making might play out in those domains. We suggest utilizing these samples in building learning opportunities following each of the core topics.

Z. D. Berger
Division of General Internal Medicine, Department of Medicine, John Hopkins School of Medicine, Baltimore, MD, USA
e-mail: zberger1@jhmi.edu

D. R. Nandiwada
Division of General Internal Medicine, Department of Medicine, Penn Center for Primary Care Penn Presbyterian Hospital, University of Pennsylvania Perelman School of Medicine, Philadelphia, PA, USA
e-mail: deepa.nandiwada@pennmedicine.upenn.edu

D. A. Zipkin (✉)
Department of Medicine, Duke University Health System, Duke University School of Medicine, Durham, NC, USA
e-mail: daniella.zipkin@duke.edu

D. A. Zipkin (ed.), *Teaching Evidence-Based Medicine*,
https://doi.org/10.1007/978-3-031-11174-7_11

Introduction

Shared decision making is not an algorithm but a model of relationships between doctors and patients. As the clinician, you seek to empower the patient to make their own decisions, helping them understand and fulfill their role in a way that is appropriate for them [1]. In this way, the physician is like the front-seat passenger in a truck. The clinician guides the patient, but the patient is driving.

At the same time, the patient's comfort and preferences for participation in decision making should be assessed; for example, some patients might prefer decisions to be made by the physician [2]. Care should be taken not to assume such preferences. Finally, shared decision making should allow the patient to say no to any therapeutic, diagnostic, or other clinical decision, without fear of abandonment [3].

Shared decision making can take different forms in different circumstances. However, at the extremes, such as treatments that are the gold standard or ineffective therapies, shared decision making does not apply in the strictest sense. A treatment recognized as effective in a situation where some intervention is considered necessary might not require a full range of shared decision making practices, for example, acute sepsis is not generally accompanied by a detailed discussion with patients of the risks and benefits of fluid supplementation. Similarly, in the other direction, testing copper levels as part of diagnostic workup for pain is neither broadly recommended nor based in any notion of evidence and therefore is not a topic to bring up through shared decision making [4].

Treatments or testing which are the topic of dispute and discussion are perfect topics for shared decision making, e.g., prescribing a statin for primary prevention of coronary artery disease. Most effective therapies have been shown to reduce morbidity or delay mortality to some degree, but by and large they do not totally eliminate morbidity, and they typically have some potential harms. Most day to day clinical decisions involve a balance of benefits and harms, and ideally we would tailor those estimates to the patient whenever their specific risks are known. In addition, many things which are widely considered good medicine may still be declined by a patient, (e.g., insulin for refractory diabetes); helping patients make their own decision means acquiescing in decisions you disagree with. By the same token, you are expected and allowed to share your opinion. While the final decision belongs to the patient, you are a clinician (or a clinician in training) and should advocate for what you see as the best decision if the patient asks [5].

What follows are our recommended steps in carrying out shared decision making in clinical settings.

Develop a Script

Shared decision making is not just an ideology but a practice. You need to develop a "script" for engaging in shared decision making on a particular topic, much as you have other scripts for common clinical situations. For example, when you discuss taking a statin, the question is not necessarily merely "do you want to take a statin or not," but "how do you understand the significance of the long-term risk for cardiovascular disease, and the imperfect evidence regarding statins and primary prevention?" Such scripts should include your understanding about the evidence and guidelines and a transparent statement about your practice style, bias, and interpretation of that evidence.

Assess the Patient's Context

Next, you should assess your patient's personal context regarding the clinical topic. What are their preferences and concerns regarding the clinical condition and the options for treatment, diagnosis, or palliation? What barriers such as cost, accessibility, time, and transportation are relevant to them [6]? Are there family members who might have been affected or should be involved in the decision? More broadly, consider the social context of the clinical topic in question. Conditions like cancer, chronic pain, and depression—in fact, all clinical entities—are connected to cultural, political, and social phenomena which clinicians should be aware of in the context of decision making [7].

Assess Benefits and Harms

Whenever possible, assess the patient's baseline risk of the condition in question. For instance, what is the patient's risk of total cardiovascular events? Or, what is this patient's risk of stroke due to atrial fibrillation? In many cases, risk calculators are readily available, either online or integrated into electronic health records. After the baseline risk has been calculated, consider how much an intervention can reduce this risk. This process is addressed more thoroughly in Chap. 4, section "Applying and Communicating Results of Clinical Trials to Your Patient". Decision aids may help in this process, but be aware that some are biased and incomplete. Decision aids may serve as tools to further quantify and visualize benefits and harms. Displaying the impact of an intervention through bar graphs or icon arrays improves patients' understanding of their risk [8].

Assessing benefits and harms in this manner only addresses the numeric information. We must continue in the process to further integrate these numbers into shared decision making.

Integrate Patient Preferences

A patient's personal context, their preferences and concerns, should be integrated with your own recommendation. Options should be presented in patient friendly language, without coercion. Decision aids are often seen as a part of shared decision making but be aware that they are not perfect and can be inherently biased. Use them as tools to further quantify and visualize risks and benefits [9]. Further considering the example of taking a statin for primary prevention of coronary artery disease, a decision aid may present your patient with a numerically significant improvement in coronary artery disease on a statin. Even so, if a patient's preference tends otherwise (for example, perhaps she has relatives who she believes are suffering adverse events from such a medication), she may decide not to take the statin, incorporating the evidence and prioritizing her personal opinions [10].

Reach a Decision

On this basis, you should help the patient reach a decision. Consider using the teach-back method to ensure your patient has considered their decision on the basis of the preferences and concerns they expressed earlier, and that they understand how the risks and benefits line up with those preferences. The teach-back method involves asking the patient to teach the pro and cons of the clinical decision back to you to ensure that they have interpreted and understand the conversation you just had. Emphasize that decisions can be revisited, and preferences need to be iteratively reconsidered on the basis of new information, situations, and preferences. You will be there to work with them throughout, and help them turn their decisions, where appropriate, into action [11].

From Theory to Action

As noted above, shared decision making is not a dogma but a practice. The following chapters of this book will be accompanied by case vignettes and supplementary questions to help develop your shared decision making practice. Each of the above elements might be exercised in different ways, to various extents, by you and the patient given the circumstances of the case.

TEACH IT!!

This section can be used as an added teaching session in the context of a Harm exercise or a Therapy exercise. We recommend starting with a numerical assessment of benefit or harm based on the data you are working with, described in detail in Chaps. 4 and 6. For illustrative purposes, we will use the example of statins for primary prevention of cardiovascular disease, both because this is a common clinical concern in many specialties of medicine and because an excellent risk communication tool is available publicly to enhance the process. Please also see Chap. 4, section "Applying and Communicating Results of Clinical Trials to Your Patient".

15 min:

- Have learners calculate a sample patient's baseline risk of cardiovascular disease utilizing the ASCVD risk calculator. Then, present them with relative risk reduction data regarding statins for primary prevention of cardiovascular disease. Have learners estimate the absolute risk reduction for that patient.

- Armed with the absolute risk reduction, have learners attempt to speak this information to the patient.
- Using the table above, work with your learners to talk through the above steps focusing on how they would frame their shared decision-making question and what their own recommendation would be for the patient based on assessing harms and benefits.
- Have learners verbalize examples of patients' contexts and preferences which may alter the decision outcome. Discuss that the decision the patient makes may not match your own preferences and how to reconcile this!
- Ask the learners how they might visually display the absolute risk reduction to help the patient understand the true magnitude of benefit. Utilize the Mayo Clinic Statin Decision Aid, available online [12]

30 min:

- Add to the above exercise by having learners pair up. Prepare two patient scripts ahead of time, adding context and barriers of differing types to each. Have the paired teams take turns role playing being the patient in the scenario. The person in the clinician role practices how to incorporate all of the steps in shared decision making with the patient. Debrief with the group by using the table as a discussion guide.

TEACH IT!!

The sample worksheets in the appendix to this chapter can be used to complete the teaching in all of the core content domains of evidence-based medicine. We recommend filling out tables like these with your learners after the core teaching in each domain so they can develop their SDM teaching/interaction style and scripts for future use. After the table has been filled out, we recommend having learners practice scripts with each other in pairs with one individual providing counseling and the other serving as the patient.

Appendix

Shared Decision Making Worksheets

Worksheet Template

Shared decision making step	Case analysis	Example of language to be used
Triage the individual issue under discussion to deem if it is appropriate for shared decision making	What is the clinical decision?	
Develop your script for a particular topic	Frame the goal of decision making:	
Assessing your patient's personal context regarding the clinical topic	Their concerns: Barriers: Social Context:	
Assess benefits and harms	Best estimate of baseline risk: Evidence supporting risk reduction: What are the harms?	
Integrating patient context with your own recommendations	Decision Aid: Option 1: Option 2: Your recommendation: Address patient concerns:	
Reach a decision	What's the decision?	

Worksheet Example: Searching the Literature

Case: A 54-year-old woman who had chronic right knee osteoarthritis and interested in getting a steroid knee injection.

SDM step	Case analysis	Example of language to be used
Triaging the individual issue under discussion to deem if it is appropriate for SDM	What is the clinical decision?	What is the effectiveness of steroid injection in the treatment of knee pain from osteoarthritis? (Search for a decision aid, or, if one is lacking, a guideline or useful evidence-based resource to assist.)
Developing your SDM script for a particular topic	What is your goal: What is the evidence: What is your preference:	
Assessing your patient's personal context regarding the clinical topic	What is their preference: Their concerns: Barriers: Social Context:	They would like relief of pain. They are worried about side effects but are not opposed to injection. No significant barriers. She is able to make it to an appointment for an injection and could afford it.
Assess Benefits and Harms	Best estimate of baseline risk: N/A Evidence supporting risk reduction: N/A Evidence supporting benefit: What are the harms?	
Integrating patient context with your own recommendations	Decision Aid/EBM resources: Option 1: Option 2: Your recommendation: Address patient concerns:	
Reach a decision	What's the decision?	

Worksheet Example: Causation/Harm

A 59-year-old man with chronic GERD comes to you wondering if he should stay on his current proton pump inhibitor that he has taken for 5 years given the reports he has read in the media about potential harms.

SDM step	Case analysis	Example of language to be used
Triaging the individual issue under discussion to deem if it is appropriate for SDM	What is the clinical decision?	Should a proton pump be continued, and how, given the evidence of potential adverse effects? (Find a decision aid, evidence-based resource, or evidence-based guideline addressing the strength of causation and how to balance harms and benefits.)
Developing your SDM script for a particular topic	What is your goal: What is the evidence: What is your preference:	
Assessing your patient's personal context regarding the clinical topic	What is their preference: Their concerns: Barriers: Social Context:	They would like relief of reflux symptoms but are worried about harms about being on a chronic medication. They are wondering whether they can take the medication on a less-than-daily basis. Social context: patient has significant anxiety about taking medications and potential harms.
Assess Benefits and Harms	Best estimate of baseline risk: Evidence supporting causation of harm: Evidence supporting benefit:	
Integrating patient context with your own recommendations	Decision Aid/EBM resources: Option 1: Option 2: Your recommendation: Address patient concerns:	
Reach a decision	What's the decision?	

Worksheet Example: Diagnosis

Your patient, 35 years old with a history of migraines, comes in requesting an MRI because of a headache which "feels different from my normal migraine." She has no focal neurological abnormalities on physical exam.

SDM step	Case analysis	Example of language to be used
Triaging the individual issue under discussion to deem if it is appropriate for SDM	What is the clinical decision?	Should MRI be pursued in a patient with a history of migraines and changed headache without neurological findings?
Developing your SDM script for a particular topic	What is your goal: What is the evidence: What is your preference:	
Assessing your patient's personal context regarding the clinical topic	What is their preference: Their concerns: Barriers: Social Context:	They would like to make sure they do not have cancer. Cost is a barrier. An aunt was diagnosed three months ago with brain cancer after headaches.
Assess Benefits and Harms	Best estimate of prevalence: Best estimate of likelihood ratios/predictive values/NNT: What are the harms?	
Integrating patient context with your own recommendations	Decision Aid/EBM resources: Option 1: Option 2: Your recommendation: Address patient concerns:	
Reach a decision	What's the decision?	

Worksheet Example: Screening

A 60-year-old Spanish-speaking man with a 30-pack-year smoking history, who quit smoking 5 years ago, asks you whether he should get the "lung cancer test." He is asymptomatic.

SDM step	Case analysis	Example of language to be used
Triaging the individual issue under discussion to deem if it is appropriate for SDM	What is the clinical decision?	Is this patient eligible for lung cancer screening per evidence-based guidelines? If he is eligible, what is the benefit to him of screening, and should he be screened?
Developing your SDM script for a particular topic	What is your goal: What is the evidence: What is your preference:	
Assessing your patient's personal context regarding the clinical topic	What is their preference: Their concerns: Barriers: Social Context:	"I would like to do whatever you recommend, doctor." He is concerned about cancer. Cost is a barrier. You have seen him before. His health literacy is poor in Spanish and English.
Assess Benefits and Harms	Best estimate of baseline risk: Evidence supporting risk reduction: Evidence supporting benefit: Evidence regarding test characteristics: What are the harms?	
Integrating patient context with your own recommendations	Decision Aid/EBM resources: Option 1: Option 2: Your recommendation: Address patient concerns:	
Reach a decision	What's the decision?	

Worksheet Example: Therapy

A 45-year-old woman with chronic back pain, fatigue, decreased energy, and anhedonia has been recently diagnosed by you with depression and returns to discuss treatment options. Her PHQ-9 is 15. She is able to work and be active in home life but finds her symptoms very disruptive; they keep her from playing with her kids as she would like to. She often feels overwhelmed. She has no suicidal ideation.

SDM step	Case analysis	Example of language to be used
Triaging the individual issue under discussion to deem if it is appropriate for SDM	What is the clinical decision?	Is psychotherapy, pharmacotherapy, or both the most appropriate option? If medication is indicated, which would you and she choose? (Find a guideline and/or evidence-based resource comparing pharmacotherapy and psychotherapy.)
Developing your SDM script for a particular topic	What is your goal: What is the evidence: What is your preference:	
Assessing your patient's personal context regarding the clinical topic	What is their preference: Their concerns: Barriers: Social Context:	She is wary of the side effects of medications and has never tried psychotherapy before. She is worried that she will have to be a on a habit-forming medication for the rest of her life. Barriers: There are only a few psychotherapists taking new patients who accept her insurance. Time commitment for weekly visits is also difficult given childcare and work.
Assess Benefits and Harms	Evidence supporting benefit of pharma Evidence supporting benefit of psychotherapy What are the harms?	
Integrating patient context with your own recommendations	Decision Aid/EBM resources: Option 1: Option 2: Your recommendation: Address patient concerns:	
Reach a decision	What's the decision?	

Worksheet Example: Prognosis

A 65-year-old grandmother comes to you to discuss her worsening shortness of breath. She has severe COPD (GOLD stage D) without significant comorbidities; she quit tobacco 15 years ago. She would like to know what she can expect for the future. She is on home oxygen and has been hospitalized three times in the past year. She is on a long acting beta agonist, inhaled corticosteroid, anticholinergic, and daily prednisone 10 mg. She likes to chat with her grandchildren and can walk to the kitchen and bathroom on the first floor of her house.

SDM step	Case analysis	Example of language to be used
Triaging the individual issue under discussion to deem if it is appropriate for SDM	What is the clinical decision?	What is the prognosis, both regarding life expectancy and quality of life, associated with this patient's severe COPD? What should be the approach to her care on that basis? (Search for an evidence-based guideline regarding the prognosis of patients with severe COPD, including medical and surgical options.)
Developing your SDM script for a particular topic	What is your goal: What is the evidence: What is your preference:	
Assessing your patient's personal context regarding the clinical topic	What is their preference: Their concerns: Barriers: Social Context:	She would like to remain as active as possible and maximize her time with her grandchildren. She wonders whether there is any possibility of lung transplant but worries about risk of surgery. Cost is not a barrier. She has good social support.
Assess Benefits and Harms	Evidence supporting benefit of transplant compared to continue medical therapy Evidence regarding prognosis of severe COPD (life expectancy, quality of life) What are the harms?	
Integrating patient context with your own recommendations	Decision Aid/EBM resources: Option 1: Option 2: Your recommendation: Address patient concerns:	
Reach a decision	What's the decision?	

Worksheet Example: Systematic Reviews

A 45-year-old working mother of three is healthy and without symptoms. She recently heard about two friends diagnosed with cancer and would like to know how best to prevent cancer. She wonders if there are foods she should include or avoid in her diet. She knows there have been a number of scientific studies—she has read about them in the lay press—but finds their results contradictory and confusing.

SDM step	Case analysis	Example of language to be used
Triaging the individual issue under discussion to deem if it is appropriate for SDM	What is the clinical decision?	What cancer-preventing diet, if any, should be recommended to this healthy patient? (Seek evidence-based resources regarding diet and cancer.)
Developing your SDM script for a particular topic	What is your goal: What is the evidence: What is your preference:	
Assessing your patient's personal context regarding the clinical topic	What is their preference: Their concerns: Barriers: Social Context:	She would like to reduce her risk of cancer. She enjoys a variety of foods but cost is a barrier. Her health literacy is high.
Assess Benefits and Harms	Evidence regarding absolute and relative risk reduction of diet in cancer What are the harms of pursuing specific diets?	
Integrating patient context with your own recommendations	Decision Aid/EBM resources: Option 1: Option 2: Your recommendation: Address patient concerns:	
Reach a decision	What's the decision?	

Worksheet Example: Non-inferiority

Your 66-year-old patient has atrial fibrillation and hypertension without other comorbidities. He enjoys building useful objects out of wood. He has been taking warfarin for years without noticeable adverse effects and has read about "new blood thinners." He wonders if he should switch.

SDM step	Case analysis	Example of language to be used
Triaging the individual issue under discussion to deem if it is appropriate for SDM	What is the clinical decision?	Should this patient change from warfarin to a direct oral anticoagulant (DOAC)? Is a DOAC noninferior to warfarin for this patient? (Ascertain an evidence-based source to answer this question.)
Developing your SDM script for a particular topic	What is your goal: What is the evidence: What is your preference:	
Assessing your patient's personal context regarding the clinical topic	What is their preference: Their concerns: Barriers: Social Context:	Cost is a barrier but he finds it inconvenient to go to the anticoagulation clinic sometimes multiple times a week. He is concerned about avoiding bleeding.
Assess Benefits and Harms	Evidence regarding noninferiority of DOACs compared to warfarin. Evidence comparing the harms.	
Integrating patient context with your own recommendations	Decision Aid/EBM resources: Option 1: Option 2: Your recommendation: Address patient concerns:	
Reach a decision	What's the decision?	

Worksheet Example: Learner Assessment

This format can also be valuable in assessing your learners' performance within evidence-based practice. What to look for from learners for each topic:

SDM step	Case analysis	What to look for in your learners
Triaging the individual issue under discussion to deem if it is appropriate for SDM	What is the clinical decision?	Can they develop a PICO question to search the literature
Developing your SDM script for a particular topic	What is your goal: What is the evidence: What is your preference:	Are they able to interpret the evidence to commit to what their own recommendation/preference would be?
Assessing your patient's personal context regarding the clinical topic	What is their preference: Their concerns: Barriers: Social Context:	Are they able to integrate social context and barriers into the script they develop to speak with the patient while practicing role plays at the end?
Assess Benefits and Harms	Evidence supporting benefit of transplant compared to continue medical therapy Evidence regarding prognosis of severe COPD (life expectancy, quality of life) What are the harms?	
Integrating patient context with your own recommendations	Decision Aid/EBM resources: Option 1: Option 2: Your recommendation: Address patient concerns:	How actively does the learner include the patient in the discussion and use of a decision aid. Are they able to troubleshoot the patient's concerns using the evidence. Do they avoid jargon. Do they explain the statistics in patient friendly language?
Reach a decision	What's the decision?	

References

1. Charles C, Gafni A, Whelan T. Decision-making in the physician–patient encounter: revisiting the shared treatment decision-making model. Soc Sci Med. 1999;49(5):651–61.
2. Cribb A, Entwistle VA. Shared decision making: trade-offs between narrower and broader conceptions. Health Expect. 2011;14(2):210–9.
3. LM O. Stop the silent misdiagnosis patients' preferences matter. BMJ. 2012;345:23.
4. Berger ZD, Brito JP, Ospina NS, Kannan S, Hinson JS, Hess EP, Haskell H, Montori VM, Newman-Toker DE. Patient centred diagnosis: sharing diagnostic decisions with patients in clinical practice. BMJ. 2017;359:j4218.
5. Brock DW. The ideal of shared decision making between physicians and patients. Kennedy Inst Ethics J. 1991;1(1):28–47.
6. Joseph-Williams N, Elwyn G, Edwards A. Knowledge is not power for patients: a systematic review and thematic synthesis of patient-reported barriers and facilitators to shared decision making. Patient Educ Couns. 2014;94(3):291–309.
7. Peek ME, Odoms-Young A, Quinn MT, Gorawara-Bhat R, Wilson SC, Chin MH. Race and shared decision-making: perspectives of African-Americans with diabetes. Soc Sci Med. 2010;71(1):1–9.
8. Zipkin DA, Umscheid CA, et al. Evidence-based risk communication: a systematic review. 733 Ann Intern Med. 2014;161:270–80.
9. Agoritsas T, Heen AF, Brandt L, Alonso-Coello P, Kristiansen A, Akl EA, Neumann I, Tikkinen KAO, van der Weijden T, Elwyn G, Montori VM, Guyatt GH, Vandvik PO. Decision aids that really promote shared decision making: the pace quickens. BMJ. 2015;350:g7624.
10. Elwyn G, Frosch D, Thomson R, Joseph-Williams N, Lloyd A, Kinnersley P, Cording E, Tomson D, Dodd C, Rollnick S, Edwards A. Shared decision making: a model for clinical practice. J Gen Intern Med. 2012;27(10):1361–7.
11. Hoffmann TC, Légaré F, Simmons MB, McNamara K, McCaffery K, Trevena LJ, Hudson B, Glasziou PP, Del Mar CB. Shared decision making: what do clinicians need to know and why should they bother? Med J Aust. 2014;201(1):35–9.
12. https://statindecisionaid.mayoclinic.org. Accessed 15 June 2021.

Index

D. A. Zipkin (ed.), *Teaching Evidence-Based Medicine*,
https://doi.org/10.1007/978-3-031-11174-7

MIX
Papier aus verantwortungsvollen Quellen
Paper from responsible sources
FSC® C105338

If you have any concerns about our products,
you can contact us on
ProductSafety@springernature.com

In case Publisher is established outside the EU,
the EU authorized representative is:
Springer Nature Customer Service Center GmbH
Europaplatz 3, 69115 Heidelberg, Germany

Printed by Libri Plureos GmbH
in Hamburg, Germany